Program Implementation in Preventive Trials

Program Implementation in Preventive Trials has been co-published simultaneously as *Journal of Prevention & Intervention in the Community*, Volume 17, Number 2 1998.

The *Journal of Prevention & Intervention in the Community* Monographs/ "Separates"
(formerly the *Prevention in Human Services* series)*

Families as Nurturing Systems: Support Across the Life Span, edited by Donald G. Unger and Douglas R. Powell*

Religion and Prevention in Mental Health: Research, Vision, and Action, edited by Kenneth I. Pargament, Kenneth I. Maton, and Robert E. Hess*

Prevention and School Transitions, edited by Leonard A. Jason, Karen E. Danner, and Karen S. Kurasaki*

Self-Help and Mutual Aid Groups: International and Multicultural Perspectives, edited by Francine Lavoie, Thomasina Borkman, and Benjamin Gidron*

International Approaches to Prevention in Mental Health and Human Services, edited by Robert E. Hess and Wolfgang Stark*

Sexual Assault and Abuse: Sociocultural Context of Prevention, edited by Carolyn F. Swift*

Preventing Illness Among People with Coronary Heart Disease, edited by John D. Piette, Robert M. Kaplan, and Joseph R. Ferrari

Adolescent Health Care: Program Designs and Services, edited by John S. Wodarski, Marvin D. Feit, and Joseph R. Ferrari

Education in Community Psychology: Models for Graduate and Undergraduate Programs, edited by Clifford R. O'Donnell and Joseph R. Ferrari

Diversity Within the Homeless Population: Implications for Intervention, edited by Elizabeth M. Smith and Joseph R. Ferrari

Manhood Development in Urban African-American Communities, edited by Roderick J. Watts and Robert J. Jagers

Preventing Drunk Driving, edited by Elsie R. Shore and Joseph R. Ferrari

Program Implementation in Preventive Trials, edited by Joseph A. Durlak and Joseph R. Ferrari

For information on previous issues of *Prevention in Human Services*, edited by Robert E. Hess.

Program Implementation in Preventive Trials

Joseph A. Durlak
Joseph R. Ferrari
Editors

Program Implementation in Preventive Trials has been co-published simultaneously as *Journal of Prevention & Intervention in the Community*, Volume 17, Number 2 1998.

Routledge
Taylor & Francis Group
NEW YORK AND LONDON

Program Implementation in Preventive Trials has been co-published simultaneously as *Journal of Prevention & Intervention in the Community*, Volume 17, Number 2 1998.

First published 1998 by
The Haworth Press, Inc.

Published 2013 by Routledge
605 Third Avenue, New York, NY 10017
4 Park Square, Milton Park, Abingdon, Oxon OX14 4RN

Routledge is an imprint of the Taylor & Francis Group, an informa business

Cover design by Thomas J. Mayshock Jr.

Library of Congress Cataloging-in-Publication Data

Program implementation in preventive trials / Joseph A. Durlak, Joseph R. Ferrari, editors
p. cm.
"Has been co-published simultaneously as Journal of prevention & intervention in the community, volume 17, number 2, 1998."
Includes bibliographical references and index.
ISBN 0-7890-0523-9
ISBN 978-0-789-00523-6 (hbk)
1. Child psychopathology–Prevention. 2. Adolescent psychopathology–Prevention. 3. Juvenile delinquency–Prevention. 4. Community psychology. I. Durlak, Joseph A. II. Ferrari, Joseph R. III. Journal of prevention & intervention in the community.
RJ499.P716 1998
618.92′8905–dc21

98-3323
CIP

ISBN 13: 978-0-7890-0523-6 (hbk)

Program Implementation in Preventive Trials

CONTENTS

ABOUT THE EDITORS

Joseph A. Durlak, PhD, Guest Editor, is Professor of Psychology at Loyola University in Chicago, Illinois. He was previously on the faculty at Southern Illinois University in Carbondale and a clinical psychologist in the U.S. Army. His main research interests in community psychology are in prevention and school-based interventions. He has published two books on prevention: *School-Based Prevention Programs for Children and Adolescents* (Sage) and *Successful Prevention Programs for Children and Adolescents* (Plenum).

Joseph R. Ferrari, PhD, is Associate Professor in the Department of Psychology at DePaul University in Chicago, Illinois, and Editor-in-Chief of the *Journal of Prevention & Intervention in the Community* since 1995. Dr. Ferrari received his PhD from Adelphi University, with a concentration in experimental social-personality psychology. In addition to his interest in mainstream social psychological issues, such as persuasion, attribution theory, and altruism, he has developed several lines of research in social-community psychology. His community research includes the psychological sense of community, caregiver stress and satisfaction, volunteerism and community service, and behavior analysis applications to community issues.

Why Worry About Implementation Procedures: Why Not Just Do?

Joseph R. Ferrari
DePaul University

Joseph A. Durlak
Loyola University

At the base of community psychology is the premise of "action." As a discipline, community psychology focuses on the development of interventions designed for the masses, utilizing varied, existing resources for program development (Kelly, 1971). Much of the research in the field is empirically driven, as opposed to a strong emphasis on developing abstract theories. In other words, community psychologists emphasize creating programs that address societal problems by developing interventions for the field, not the lab (Levine & Perkins, 1987). In fact, the notion of "doing ecological good" as opposed to "watching from the sidelines" may be a reason that attracts so many gifted professionals to the field of community psychology.

This present volume calls attention to the need for assessing *implementation*. Community programs should be comprehensively evaluated. Before we begin making any conclusions about a program's impact, we need to understand how the intervention was conducted. There can be quite a difference between what is planned and what actually happens in community-based programs. Monitoring implementation procedures in

[Haworth co-indexing entry note]: "Why Worry About Implementation Procedures: Why Not Just Do?" Ferrari, Joseph R., and Joseph A. Durlak. Co-published simultaneously in *Journal of Prevention & Intervention in the Community* (The Haworth Press, Inc.) Vol. 17, No. 2, 1998, pp. 1-3; and: *Program Implementation in Preventive Trials* (ed: Joseph A. Durlak, and Joseph R. Ferrari) The Haworth Press, Inc., 1998, pp. 1-3. Single or multiple copies of this article are available for a fee from The Haworth Document Delivery Service [1-800-342-9678, 9:00 a.m. - 5:00 p.m. (EST). E-mail address: getinfo@haworthpressinc.com].

field research is the equivalent of manipulation checks in laboratory studies–a concern over how well and effective the intervention (or, independent variable) was introduced in the study.

The concept of implementation means more than program evaluation; it includes program adherence. As the articles in this volume demonstrate, there is a need for constant monitoring of a program's continued utilization. Questions to be addressed include: Does the current setting personnel follow the implementation program? Will new members to the setting understand and utilize the procedures developed for that setting? Will the procedures be modified such that their utility decreases? These and other issues plague community psychologists interested in establishing programs of change in settings that facilitate the lives of others.

The articles in this volume give excellent examples of community-based research that focus on implementation. We begin with a paper by one of the co-editors (Durlak) in which the need for studying implementation programs is presented. Durlak stresses that when investigators have examined implementation, they often find that implementation is far from perfect and can be seriously deficient. Additional research indicates that the level of implementation achieved in community-based interventions influences outcomes. We obviously need more research on the factors that affect program implementation. He also offers useful, constructive guidelines for ways to ensure that intervention programs are conducted as planned. The following articles demonstrate effective use of those guidelines with children, adolescents, and adults (e.g., parents and teachers), and with target issues including alcohol use, substance abuse, mental health, and inner-city violence. Taken together, these articles show how necessary it is to collect implementation data in community-based research.

Briefly, we would like to highlight some of the important points made by the authors included in this volume. For instance, Clarke covers the important role of *protocol compliance* in treatment programs, particularly in mental health treatment. Defined as the degree to which interventions follow written instructions or guidelines found in manuals and other sources, protocol compliance is crucial for a program. Williams and Perry highlight the importance of flexibility so necessary modifications can be made in program procedures. By targeting the team members who "buy-in" to the intervention program (and thereby including a *multi-change agent approach*, such as parents and teachers), it is possible to enhance program adherence. Lynch, Geller, Hunt, Galano, and Dubas provide several ways in which to *enhance implementation* in a program targeted for young children. For instance, the use of data from implementation measures can provide ongoing performance feedback to the change agents in the setting. Hines, Macias, and Perrino raise the very important issue of *cultural sensitivity*: programs are more likely to be adopted and faithfully conducted in communities when program features relating to values, norms, and language are ecologically congruent with the local setting and its inhabitants. Durlak and Ferrari end this special volume by discussing some exemplars in program implementation and offer questions to guide future research. Taken together, these articles illustrate that studying implementation is a necessary part of program evaluation.

In conclusion, we think implementation should be a fundamental issue for scholars and students interested in community research and action. The questions raised and the positive examples provided should be helpful for anyone who wishes to enhance their program agenda. We acknowledge that implementation research has further to go before the final word is spoken. Nevertheless, we hope that this volume will bring the importance of implementation to the attention of community-based researchers and advocates.

REFERENCES

Kelly, J. (1971). Qualities for the community psychologist. *American Psychologist, 26*, 897-903.

Levine, M., & Perkins, D.V. (1987). *Principles of Community Psychology: Perspectives and Applications*. New York: Oxford University Press.

Why Program Implementation Is Important

Joseph A. Durlak
Loyola University Chicago

SUMMARY. Program implementation refers to how well a proposed program or intervention is put into practice and is fundamental to establishing the internal, external, construct, and statistical conclusion validity of outcome evaluations. Research conducted on preventive field trials indicates that program implementation is variable across change agents and settings and is sometimes seriously compromised, and that the level of implementation influences outcomes. Preventionists should not expect that the quantity or quality of program implementation will be a perfect 100%. Four major steps in studying implementation are discussed and suggestions are offered to insure better levels of implementation. *[Article copies available for a fee from The Haworth Document Delivery Service: 1-800-342-9678. E-mail address: getinfo@haworth.com]*

Implementation refers to how well a proposed program or intervention is put into practice and has been alternatively referred to as treatment adherence, fidelity or integrity, or sometimes, as one form of process research or process evaluation. Implementation can be distinguished from other aspects of program diffusion such as dissemination (efforts to inform others of the existence of a program and its findings); adoption (a specific decision to initiate a program) and maintenance or institutionalization (the continuation of a program after its trial adoption).

Address correspondence to: Joseph A. Durlak, Department of Psychology, Loyola University Chicago, 6525 North Sheridan Road, Chicago, IL 60626.

[Haworth co-indexing entry note]: "Why Program Implementation Is Important." Durlak, Joseph A. Co-published simultaneously in *Journal of Prevention & Intervention in the Community* (The Haworth Press, Inc.) Vol. 17, No. 2, 1998, pp. 5-18; and: *Program Implementation in Preventive Trials* (ed: Joseph A. Durlak, and Joseph R. Ferrari) The Haworth Press, Inc., 1998, pp. 5-18. Single or multiple copies of this article are available for a fee from The Haworth Document Delivery Service [1-800-342-9678, 9:00 a.m. - 5:00 p.m. (EST). E-mail address: getinfo@haworthpressinc.com].

Implementation has been relatively neglected in outcome research. Reviews covering over 1,000 *treatment* studies (Gresham, Gansle & Noell, 1993; Gresham, Gansle, Noell, Cohen & Rosenblum, 1993; Moncher & Prinz, 1991; Peterson, Homer & Wonderlich, 1982) indicate that only a small proportion of researchers (between 14% to 24%) check carefully to see how well therapists adhere to treatment protocols. Less than 5% of over 1200 published prevention studies provide data on program implementation (Durlak, 1997). The intent of this paper is to stress the fundamental importance of program implementation, review representative research in prevention, outline the steps involved in studying implementation, and offer a few suggestions about insuring better levels of implementation.

IMPORTANCE OF IMPLEMENTATION

Information on implementation is critical to the validity of program evaluations. We cannot make confident connections between programs and outcomes (internal validity), expect to replicate interventions in other settings (external validity), or determine how or why a program works (construct validity) without knowing how well the proposed program was actually conducted. Statistical conclusion validity can also be affected because variability in implementation introduces error variance that reduces the power of statistical analyses.

Implementation data are critical for interpreting both positive and negative results. In the former case, we cannot attribute positive findings to a program unless we know if the program in question was actually conducted. Suppose investigators used a dismantling design in order to assess the influence of adding different components to a program and found that those who received only component A improved just as much as those who received components A plus B, or components A plus B plus C. The temptation is to assume that only element A is necessary for change and the other components are superfluous; however, such findings might result if A was the only component that was faithfully implemented. If components B or C, or both, were well-executed, they might substantially increase program effects.

If negative results occur and implementation is not monitored, there is the danger that some potentially useful programs will be prematurely and unfairly rejected for the wrong reasons. Nonsignificant findings can result when a potentially powerful program is poorly implemented and thus never put to a fair test. Assessing implementation is so crucial that the term *Type III error* has been coined in reference to program evaluations that fail to consider implementation (Scanlon, Horst, Nay, Schmidt, & Waller,

1977). Unless we assess implementation, we do not really know what we are evaluating and are making a Type III error.

Implementation is important at every stage of research from initial pilot studies to large-scale field trials, but the focus of this paper is on effectiveness as opposed to efficacy trials. Although efficacy and effectiveness trials are not mutually exclusive, the former refers to research done under carefully controlled situations, while effectiveness trials are a test of intervention impact in real world settings. Implementation is likely to be better in efficacy trials (although this assumption should be empirically assessed), because investigators can exercise stronger experimental control over such factors as the identity, training and supervision of change agents, recruitment and selection of the target population and the conduct of outcome assessments. In effectiveness trials, however, the program is offered by staff or volunteers in field-based settings who are often learning new procedures for the first time and have many other demands on their time in addition to implementing a new program.

DEFINING IMPLEMENTATION

Implementation is not an all-or-none construct but exists in degrees along a continuum, from 0% to 100%. Throughout this paper, the referent in implementation is to the active ingredients of an innovation, that is, those elements believed to be responsible for a program's effects. There will always be some variation across settings in how programs are conducted, and there is growing recognition that interventions must be tailored to fit local conditions (Elias, 1997; Meyer, Miller & Herman, 1993). The concern in implementation then is how well the program's active ingredients are delivered although whatever tailoring or modifying that is done to the intervention should be described to guide others wishing to adapt the program to their setting.

RESEARCH ON IMPLEMENTATION

Prevention research offers two clear conclusions regarding implementation: (1) implementation is variable across change agents and settings and is sometimes seriously compromised; and (2) level of implementation influences outcomes.

Implementation Is Variable. Table 1 summarizes the results of representative field studies on the level of implementation attained in different

TABLE 1. Prevention Studies Illustrating How Implementation Can Be Compromised

Study	Reflection of Low or Poor Implementation
Battistich, Schaps, Watson & Solomon (1996)	Implementation of a system-level intervention was poor in 4 of 12 schools (33%)
Bush et al. (1989)	No teacher conducted a proposed program as planned, either quantitatively or qualitatively
Flannery & Torquati (1993)	67% of teachers failed to implement a key program component
Rohrbach, Graham & Hansen (1993)	79% of teachers omitted program components
Taggart, Bush, Zuckerman & Theiss (1990)	Only 46% of teachers implemented a program effectively
Tobler (1986)	26% of 143 drug prevention programs were improperly implemented
Tortu & Botvin (1989)	Teachers omitted between 25% to 54% of program activities
Wall, Severson, Andrews, Lichenstein & Zoref (1995)	Staff omitted between 27% to 81% of program activities

prevention programs. Between 23% to 81% of program activities may be omitted (Smith et al., 1993; Wall et al., 1995), and only a minority of change agents may implement the program with a high degree of integrity or fidelity (e.g., Bush et al., 1989; Taggart et al., 1990). As a general rule, preventionists should not expect that the quantity or quality of implementation will be 100%. At the same time, we do not know what level of implementation is necessary for maximum program impact and what levels are feasible under different circumstances.

Implementation Affects Outcomes. Results from several studies examining the connection between implementation and outcome are summarized in Table 2. These data suggest two general findings: (1) for some programs positive effects occur only when a certain level of implementation is attained; and (2) for other programs better or higher levels of implementation are associated with stronger or more positive outcomes. For instance, Connell, Turner and Mason (1985) found that two of the four health education programs they examined had to be implemented for at least 20 hours and include parents as the program model specified in order

TABLE 2. Prevention Studies Linking Implementation to Outcomes

Study	Type/Goal of Program	General Findings
Battistich, Schaps, Watson & Solomon (1996)	Improve school practices, organization, climate	Only well-implemented programs had positive effects
Botvin, Baker, Dusenbury, Botvin, & Diaz (1995)	drug prevention	Better implementation associated with stronger effects
Botvin, Dusenbury, Baker, James-Ortiz & Kerner (1989)	drug prevention	Only well-implemented programs had positive effects
Bush et al. (1989)	health education	Better implementation associated with stronger effects
Connell, Turner & Mason (1985)	health education	Better implementation associated with stronger effects
Greenwood, Terry, Arreaga-Mayer & Finney (1992)	classwide peer tutoring	Better implementation associated with stronger effects
Hansen, Graham, Wolkenstein & Rohrbach (1991)	alcohol prevention	Better implementation associated with stronger effects
McGraw et al. (1996)	CATCH: school-based health education	Better implementation predicted better outcomes
Pentz et al. (1990)	drug prevention	Only well-implemented programs had positive effects
Ross, Luepker, Nelson, Saavedra & Hubbard (1991)	high school health education	Only well-implemented programs had positive effects
Taggart, Bush, Zuckerman & Theiss (1990)	Know Your Body health education program	Only well-implemented programs had positive effects
Tobler (1986)	review of 143 drug prevention studies	Well-implemented programs achieved effect sizes 0.34 greater than poorly-implemented programs

to produce a significant positive effect. Three other studies have found that poorly implemented prevention programs were not successful (Botvin et al., 1989; Ross et al., 1991; Taggart et al., 1990).

Information from additional studies indicates how outcomes improve as implementation improves. In Botvin et al.'s (1995) evaluation of a school-based drug prevention program, analyses involving the total study sample indicated that rates of cigarette smoking were significantly lower (by 21%) for the experimental group than the controls, but there were no significant differences between groups for either alcohol or marijuana use. However, among those students whose teachers were considered to have implemented the program with good integrity, significant differences favoring the experimental over the control group occurred for all three drugs: tobacco (27% less), alcohol (24% less) and marijuana use (21% less). In summary, this program was much more effective when it was properly conducted.

A similar finding occurred for the Midwestern Prevention Project, another drug prevention program (Pentz et al., 1990). The investigators analyzed results separately for students in 12 program schools in which the level of implementation was high and 12 other program schools in which level of implementation was low. Students in low implementation schools demonstrated approximately 18% less cigarette smoking, 25% less alcohol use, and virtually the same level of marijuana use as controls. In this case, even low levels of implementation yielded some positive benefits, but stronger effects were found among students in high implementation schools. These students demonstrated approximately 43% less cigarette smoking, 34% less alcohol use, and 33% less marijuana use than controls. In separate comparisons with controls, students in the high implementation schools had over 2 and one-half less drug use than those in the low implementation schools.

Tobler's (1986) meta-analysis of drug prevention programs also reflects how implementation moderates outcomes. Well-implemented programs achieved a mean effect size 0.34 greater than poorly implemented programs. The magnitude of this difference is substantial because all 143 programs reviewed by Tobler (1986) attained an overall mean effect of only 0.30. Finally, the power of implementation in affecting outcome was shown in a regression analysis for a health education program designed to change children's dietary habits. McGraw et al. (1996) found that each 1% increase in teachers' level of implementation accounted for a 10% increase in their students' self-report efficacy in selecting healthy foods.

In summary, research clearly indicates the importance of program implementation: the level of implementation influences outcomes and poor implementation can jeopardize program impact. Because implementation data are crucial but are rarely collected, the next section describes some procedures for studying implementation.

STEPS IN STUDYING IMPLEMENTATION

There are four major steps involved in studying implementation: (1) defining active program ingredients; (2) developing an accurate and valid assessment system; (3) monitoring implementation during program execution; and (4) relating implementation levels to outcomes.

Step 1: Define Active Program Ingredients

The first step involves using theory or past research to define the program's active ingredients in clear operational terms. Interventions should be guided by beliefs explaining why they should work. These beliefs generally determine the number and often the sequence of program components. The law of parsimony stresses the value of simplicity. Therefore, the ideal program contains no more elements than are needed to achieve desired goals and is provided in sufficient dosage or intensity to achieve its intended effect.

The most common way to translate active program ingredients into practice is through the use of program manuals which establish a detailed protocol for the intervention. Manuals are designed to capture the essential components of intervention by describing what needs to be done. Some manuals insist on a very specific sequence of activities and a standardized method of delivery within each sequence including verbatim responses that change agents should practice to mastery before administering the program. Others provide general guidelines and permit greater flexibility in response and application.

Although manualized interventions are preferred by many social scientists, it is particularly difficult to specify the most appropriate interpersonal, social or cultural context for a program and to codify the interpersonal style that is preferred for different program practices. Sometimes it is not *what* but *how* something is said or done that makes a difference. These latter more subtle aspects of program delivery are difficult to prescribe in manuals and are another reason for customizing the intervention to fit the host setting and target population.

Step 2: Use Good Methods to Measure Implementation

An effective method of assessing implementation must be established. Ratings by independent observers whose reliability is assessed generally yields the most credible information. Observers can enter the setting to watch the intervention in progress or rate from video- or audiotapes. Self-reports by change agents may be the only practical way to obtain information on implementation in some situations, but the validity of these data is questionable. Inexperienced change agents may be unable to report accurately how well they conducted different aspects of a program, and self-reports are typically skewed in the positive direction (Hansen, Graham, Wolkenstein & Rohrbach, 1991; McKenzie et al., 1994). Both the quantity and the quality of implementation should be assessed. That is, we need to know how much of the program was administered and how well each part was conducted, respectively.

Step 3: Monitor Implementation

The frequency of implementation checks is important during program monitoring. Each active ingredient of a program should be assessed and multiple checks should occur over time, program components, change agents, and different program participants served by each change agent. The data are clear that levels of implementation vary across change agents involved in the same program (see Table 1), and it should not be assumed that each change agent behaves similarly with all program participants, is consistent over time and can administer each program component equally well. Program drift, which refers to significant departures from fidelity over time, can occur as change agents modify or omit program activities upon repeated administration. Data indicate that between 41% to 84% of teachers who begin preventive programs may modify them over time or discontinue their use altogether (Gingiss, Gottlieb, & Brink, 1994; Rohrbach, Graham & Hansen, 1993; Tappe, Galer-Unit & Bailey, 1995).

Collecting implementation data at multiple points increases confidence in the analysis and can be used to improve the program. After early implementation checks Greenwood et al. (1987) provided additional training to two of eight teachers who were having difficulty implementing a classroom-wide tutoring intervention.

Step 4: Relate Implementation to Outcome

The appropriate unit of analysis must be chosen to assess implementation based on the conceptual thrust of the intervention. For classroom and small group interventions the teacher or group leader is the appropriate unit of analysis, but school-wide interventions dictate that implementation data be analyzed at a school-wide level (e.g., Pentz et al., 1990). When parents are involved, methods must be developed to assess their rate and intensity of involvement. A simple grand mean to assess implementation across all change agents or settings can be misleading because it may mask the marked variability in implementation that usually occurs (see Table 1).

The data in Table 2 indicate clearly how implementation can affect outcomes if there is sufficient variability in levels of implementation. We would expect that settings in which the program is conducted very well would produce better results than settings in which implementation is poor or severely compromised. Therefore, investigators should conduct their outcome assessments so that the influence of different levels of implementation can be assessed.

What About Nonstandardized Interventions?

Some preventive interventions cannot be compartmentalized into a predetermined number and sequence of activities, such as 10, 45-minute sessions with two to three structured activities per session. Prevention is also possible through a combination of overlapping strategies involving coalition building, empowerment, capacity-building, media advocacy, social action, and participatory research (Durlak, 1997). Nevertheless, these interventions are guided by specific principles relevant to changing individuals, organizations, or communities that should suggest ways to capture the program's basic practices. With relevant theory and research as guides, different methods could be used to assess implementation that might include participant as well as independent observations, field notes, logbooks, task analyses, and personal interviews.

Neglected Aspects of Implementation

Two frequently overlooked issues in implementation involve documenting the rate and intensity of participation of the target population, and monitoring alternative programs delivered to control or comparison groups.

Target Population. Part of good program implementation involves seeing to it that eligible members from the target population participate at a reasonably high rate and intensity. In other words, did the intervention effectively attract and maintain the interest of its target population? Experience suggests that it has been easiest to involve children, teachers, and parents in prevention programs, in that order (Durlak, 1995; 1997). Children are a captive audience in school-based programs and rarely refuse to participate, although their parents might object to some aspects of sex, pregnancy, or AIDS interventions. Still, it is important to monitor children's attendance because absences, requirements to attend other school activities and family moves can lessen exposure to a program for some children. There also may be differences in participation rates in relation to grade or developmental level, social class, or ethnic group that are worth considering.

Similarly, data should be presented on the proportion of eligible school districts and teachers within each possible school who eventually participate in the program. Good implementation may be dependent on securing the participation of the most eager and committed school administrations and teaching staff rather than the typical school and teacher. This is important in judging a program's external validity. Also, when teachers vary in their initial level of motivation, this will have implications for subsequent training and consultation. Implementation is incomplete if a program is unable to attract and retain a high percentage of its target population in the intervention.

The Fantasy of Untreated Control Groups. A large majority of school districts in the United States offer multiple prevention programs covering such topics as drugs, sex, AIDS, personal safety, physical health, violence, and mental health. As a result, it may be impossible to obtain a true no-treatment control group of school children. There are three stunning examples of this point. As one example, Perry et al. (1996) reported that over 90% of those in a control condition had received an alternative drug prevention program and some had received more than one. Another research group (Ary et al., 1990) discovered that there was an alternative drug prevention program operating in 100% of control classrooms. Finally, in another study (Elder et al., 1996) one component of a multilevel intervention to affect tobacco use was to encourage schools to formulate school-wide anti-tobacco policies. Investigators found, however, that just as many control as intervention schools had developed such policies over the 3-year study period.

Therefore, evaluations of school-based programs are most likely comparing a new intervention to alternative services and the latter should be described and monitored. When two interventions are being compared, the outcomes may be only half as large in magnitude as those produced by treatment vs. no-treatment conditions (Kazdin, Bass, Ayers & Rodgers, 1990).

In effect, prevention programs often are subjected to a "double whammy" that reduces the magnitude of their impact. Imperfect levels of implementation result in the experimental group receiving less intervention than is usually assumed and the absence of true no-intervention conditions means that comparison groups are receiving more than is usually assumed. These factors should be kept in mind when judging the results of prevention, and are another reason for monitoring implementation for all those in the study sample.

SUGGESTIONS FOR IMPROVING IMPLEMENTATION

Experience suggests that several steps can be taken to improve program implementation. Eight are listed here although some have already been discussed: (1) specify the essential ingredients of an intervention; (2) collaborate with change agents in field settings to tailor the program to the target setting; (3) obtain a clear commitment to administer the agreed-upon intervention; (4) train change agents to conduct the program effectively; (5) provide on-going supervision and consultation once the program has begun; (6) be ready for unexpected problems; (7) do pilot work; and (8) designate staff with responsibilities for implementation.

Regarding point #2, collaboration with local staff to insure their meaningful input into program operations works to increase their sense of program ownership, produces a better ecological fit for the program, and generally increases administrative and technical support for the program. Organizations must be "ready" for an intervention (Elias, 1997) and among other things this means the organization is able to integrate the program into its setting and has sufficient resources such as materials, funding, time, and administrative and social support. Without collaboration with field staff, the host organization is less likely to be committed and prepared to mobilize needed resources.

Good training is critical to good implementation (point #4). Many successful programs have used a social learning training strategy, emphasized opportunities for peer collaboration and problem-solving, and provided ongoing consultation, supervision, and additional training if needed. In a social learning training approach, new skills are first defined and modeled and trainees then receive immediate systematic feedback as they practice the skills to mastery. Peer collaboration and team building exercises are used frequently in schools to allow teachers to learn from and help each other. Field staff know best what will work in their own settings and can solve many implementation problems if their expertise is sufficiently respected and they have the resources and encouragement to trouble-shoot and problem solve. Some programs have hired substitute teachers to free up time for teacher training and supervision (Elder et al., 1996), and in another program (Stevens & Slavin, 1995), the principal agreed to cover classes while teachers learned new skills.

Ongoing supervision and consultation (point #5) are often essential once the intervention begins. When it comes to implementation there is considerable truth to the dictum, "If something can go wrong, it will" (point #6). Some change agents will not be able to transfer some of their newly-learned skills successfully, or will have greater difficulty with some parts of the program than others; staff turnover, scheduling conflicts and other demands on staff time also have to be resolved. Pilot projects (point #7) are extremely helpful in debugging or fine-tuning interventions but cannot resolve all possible problems. Nevertheless, pilot work can determine if the activities related to implementation are feasible, nonintrusive, and able to capture the phenomena of interest. Finally, there should be designated staff whose primary responsibility is planning and monitoring program implementation and resolving relevant conflicts and problems (point #8). Funding agencies should allow investigators to budget for implementation staff during field trials.

In summary, research on implementation of preventive programs is in its infancy. Current information clearly indicates, however, that implementation is often variable and imperfect in field settings and that the level of implementation influences outcomes. As systematic data on implementation increase, we will become better informed about the circumstances that enhance program implementation and there should be a closer correspondence between the characteristics of prevention programs that are planned and those that are eventually conducted in real world settings.

REFERENCES

Ary, D. V., Biglan, A., Glasgow, R., Zoref, L., Black, C., Ochs, L., Severson, H., Kelly, R., Weissman, W., Lichtenstein, E., Brozovsky, P., Wirt, R., & James, L. (1990). The efficacy of social-influence prevention programs versus "standard care": Are new initiatives needed? *Journal of Behavioral Medicine, 13*, 281-296.

Battistich, V., Schaps, E., Watson, M., & Solomon, D. (1996). Prevention effects of the Child Development Project: Early findings from an ongoing multisite demonstration trial. *Journal of Adolescent Research, 11*, 12-35.

Botvin, G. J., Baker, E., Dusenbury, L., Botvin, E. M., & Diaz, T. (1995). Long-term follow-up results of a randomized drug abuse prevention trial in a white middle-class population. *Journal of the American Medical Association, 273*, 1106-1112.

Botvin, G. J., Dusenbury, L., Baker, E., James-Ortiz, S., & Kerner, J. (1989). A skills training approach to smoking prevention among Hispanic youth. *Journal of Behavioral Medicine, 12*, 279-296.

Bush, P. J., Zuckerman, A. E., Taggart, V. S., Theiss, P. K., Peleg, E. O., & Smith, S. A. (1989). Cardiovascular risk factor prevention in black school children: The "Know Your Body" evaluation project. *Health Education Quarterly, 16*, 215-227.

Connell, D. B., Turner, R. R., & Mason, E. F. (1985). Summary of findings of the school health education evaluation: Health promotion effectiveness, implementation, and costs. *Journal of School Health, 55*, 316-321.

Durlak, J. A. (1995). *School-based prevention programs for children and adolescents*. Thousand Oaks, CA: Sage.

Durlak, J. A. (1997). *Successful prevention programs for children and adolescents*. New York: Plenum Press.

Elder, J. P., Perry, C. L., Stone, E. J., Johnson, C. C., Yang, M., Edmundson, E. W., Smyth, M. H., Galati, T., Feldman, H., Cribb, P., & Parcel, G. S. (1996). Tobacco use measurement, prediction, and intervention in elementary schools in four states: The CATCH study. *Preventive Medicine, 25*, 486-494.

Elias, M. J. (1997). Reinterpreting dissemination of prevention programs as widespread implementation with effectiveness and fidelity. In R. P. Weissberg, T. P. Gullotta, R. L. Hampton, B. A. Ryan, & G. A. Adams (Eds.), *Establishing preventive services* (pp. 253-289). Thousand Oaks, CA: Sage.

Flannery, D. J., & Torquati, J. (1993). An elementary school substance abuse prevention program: Teacher and administrator perspectives. *Journal of Drug Education, 23*, 387-397.

Greenwood, C. R., Dinwiddie, G., Bailey, V., Carta, J. J., Dorsey, D., Kohler, F. W., Nelson, C., Rotholz, D., & Schulte, D. (1987). Field replication of class-wide peer tutoring. *Journal of Applied Behavior Analysis, 20*, 151-160.

Greenwood, C. R., Terry, B., Arreaga-Mayer, C., & Finney, R. (1992). The Class-wide Peer Tutoring Program: Implementation factors moderating students' achievement. *Journal of Applied Behavior Analysis, 25*, 101-116.

Gresham, F. M., Gansle, K. A., and Noell, G. H., Cohen, S., & Rosenblum, S. (1993). Treatment integrity of school-based behavioral intervention studies: 1980-1990. *School Psychology Review, 22*, 254-272.

Gresham, F. M., Gansle, K. A., & Noell, G. H. (1993). Treatment integrity in applied behavior analysis with children. *Journal of Applied Behavior Analysis, 26*, 257-263.

Hansen, W. B., Graham, J. W., Wolkenstein, B. H., & Rohrbach, L. A. (1991). Program integrity as a moderator of prevention program effectiveness: Results for fifth-grade students in the Adolescent Alcohol Prevention Trial. *Journal of Studies on Alcohol, 52*, 568-579.

Hibbs, E. D., & Jensen, P. S. (Eds.).(1996). *Psychosocial treatments for child and adolescent disorders: Empirically based strategies for clinical practice.* Washington, DC: American Psychological Association.

Kazdin, A. E., Bass, D., Ayers, W. A., & Rodgers, A. (1990). Empirical and clinical focus of child and adolescent psychotherapy research. *Journal of Consulting and Clinical Psychology, 58*, 729-740.

McGraw, S. A., Sellers, D. E., Stone, E. J., Bebchuk, J., Edmundson, E. W., Johnson, C. C., Bachman, K. J., & Luepker, R. V. (1996). Using process data to explain outcomes: An illustration from the Child and Adolescent Trial for Cardiovascular Health (CATCH). *Evaluation Review, 20*, 291-312.

Meyer, A., Miller, S., & Herman, M. (1993). Balancing the priories of evaluation with the priorities of the setting: A focus on positive youth development programs in school settings. *Journal of Primary Prevention, 14*, 95-113.

Moncher, F. J., & Prinz, R. J. (1991). Treatment fidelity in outcome studies. *Clinical Psychology Review, 11*, 247-266.

Pentz, M. A., Trebow, E. A., Hansen, W. B., MacKinnon, D. P., Dwyer, J. H., Johnson, C. A., Flay, B. R., Daniels, S., & Cormack, C. (1990). Effects of program implementation on adolescent drug use behavior: The Midwestern Prevention Project (MPP). *Evaluation Review, 14*, 264-289.

Perry, C. L., Williams, C. L., Veblen-Mortenson, S., Toomey, T. L., Komro, K. A., Anstine, P. S., McGovern, P. G., Finnegan, J. R., Forster, J. L., Wagenaar, A. C., & Wolfson, M. (1996). Outcomes of a community-wide alcohol use prevention program during early adolescence: Project Northland. *American Journal of Public Health, 86*, 956-965.

Peterson, L., Homer, A., & Wonderlich, S. (1982). The integrity of independent variables in behavior analysis. *Journal of Applied Analysis, 15*, 477-492.

Rohrbach, L. A., Graham, J. W., & Hansen, W. B. (1993). Diffusion of a school-based substance abuse prevention program: Predictors of program implementation. *Preventive Medicine, 22*, 237-260.

Ross, J. G., Luepker, R. V., Nelson, G. D., Saavedra, P., & Hubbard, B. M. (1991). Teenage health teaching modules: Impact of teacher training on implementation and student outcomes. *Journal of School Health*, *61*, 31-34.

Scanlon, J. W., Horst, P., Nay, J. N., Schmidt, R. E., & Waller, A. E. (1977) Evaluability assessment: Avoiding type III and IV errors. In G.R. Gilbert & P. J. Conklin (Eds.), *Evaluation management: A source book of readings* (pp. 71-90). Charlottesville, VA: U. S. Civil Service Commission.

Smith, D. W., McCormick, L. K., Steckler, A. B., & McLeroy, K. R. (1993). Teachers' use of health curricula: Implementation of Growing Healthy, Project SMART, and the Teenage Health Teaching Modules. *Journal of School Health*, *63*, 349-354.

Stevens, R. J., & Slavin, R. E. (1995). The cooperative elementary school: Effects on students' achievement, attitudes, and social relations. *American Educational Research Journal*, *32*, 321-351.

Taggart, V. S., Bush, P. J., Zuckerman, A. E., & Theiss, P. K. (1990). A process evaluation of the District of Columbia "Know Your Body" project. *Journal of School Health*, *60*, 60-66.

Tappe, M. K., Galer-Unti, R. A., & Bailey, K. C. (1995). Long-term implementation of the Teenage Health teaching modules by trained teachers: A case study. *Journal of School Health*, *65*, 411-415.

Tobler, N. S. (1986). Meta-analysis of 143 adolescent drug prevention programs: Quantitative outcome results of program participants compared to a control or comparison group. *Journal of Drug Issues*, *16*, 537-567.

Tortu, S., & Botvin, G. J. (1989). School-based smoking prevention: The teacher training process. *Preventive Medicine*, *18*, 280-289.

Wall, M. A., Severson, H. H., Andrews, J. A., Lichtenstein, E., & Zoref, L. (1995). Pediatric office-based smoking intervention: Impact on maternal smoking and relapse. *Pediatrics*, *96*, 622-628.

Intervention Fidelity in the Psychosocial Prevention and Treatment of Adolescent Depression

Greg Clarke
Kaiser Permanente Center for Health Research

SUMMARY. Protocol compliance, or the degree to which the delivery of mental health interventions conforms to written protocols described in manuals or outlines, is hypothesized to play an important role in mediating intervention outcomes. This paper summarizes protocol compliance assessment and data for four controlled outcome trials of adolescent depression treatment or prevention. Discussion focuses on issues pertinent to the association between fidelity and outcome, such as the unit of analysis, group versus individual interventions, the benefits and drawbacks of maximizing intervention fidelity in outcome trials, and the interaction between trial type (effectiveness vs. efficacy studies) and control over protocol compliance. *[Article copies available for a fee from The Haworth Document Delivery Service: 1-800-342-9678. E-mail address: getinfo@haworth.com]*

The past few decades have witnessed a trend towards developing of empirically-tested, manual-driven, psychosocial treatments (Hibbs & Jen-

---

Address correspondence to: Greg Clarke, Kaiser Permanente Center for Health Research, 3800 North Kaiser Center Drive, Portland, OR 97227-1098 (E-mail: clarkegr@chr.mts.kpnw.org).

This work was supported by a grant to the author (1R01-MH51318) from the Services Research Branch of the National Institute of Mental Health.

[Haworth co-indexing entry note]: "Intervention Fidelity in the Psychosocial Prevention and Treatment of Adolescent Depression." Clarke, Greg. Co-published simultaneously in *Journal of Prevention & Intervention in the Community* (The Haworth Press, Inc.) Vol. 17, No. 2, 1998, pp. 19-33; and: *Program Implementation in Preventive Trials* (ed: Joseph A. Durlak, and Joseph R. Ferrari) The Haworth Press, Inc., 1998, pp. 19-33. Single or multiple copies of this article are available for a fee from The Haworth Document Delivery Service [1-800-342-9678, 9:00 a.m. - 5:00 p.m. (EST). E-mail address: getinfo@haworthpressinc.com].

sen, 1996) and prevention programs (Durlak, this volume) for child and adolescent problem behaviors. This trend revolutionizes the study of psychosocial outcome and process in many ways. First, manuals promote dissemination of well-tested interventions, and facilitate adoption of these programs by therapists who cannot obtain direct, face-to-face training in the approach. Second, operationalizing major program components permits experimentation regarding the critical curative elements. Various sections may be compared to one another in "component analysis" to identify active elements of a particular program (e.g., Jacobson et al., 1996; Zeiss, Lewinsohn & Munoz, 1979).

Another major justification for the widespread development of intervention manuals has been to promote the consistent implementation of a program across different therapists and sites (see Clarke, 1995; Hibbs, Clarke, Hechtman, Abikoff, Greenhill & Jensen, in press), a critical issue in intervention replication and generalization. That is, is the intervention actually delivered as written, either by the originators or by subsequent adopters of the program? "Protocol compliance," "program adherence," and "treatment fidelity" all refer to how well therapists deliver the intervention as outlined in the manuals. This aspect of intervention delivery is the focus of this paper.

Significance. Typically, intervention fidelity is measured by senior clinicians who review audio- or videotaped sessions and rate the therapist's adherence to the protocol. This is distinct from subject compliance with the intervention, such as homework completion (Zimmerman, Asnis & Schwartz, 1995). From a research perspective, program fidelity is important because of the need to conduct "manipulation checks" which confirm the accurate delivery of the independent variable (in outcome trials, this is the intervention). If confirmed, differences detected between conditions can be confidently attributed to the intervention rather than to other factors. This also permits the discrimination between putatively different intervention modalities to verify that they are actually implemented in distinct fashions (e.g., Hill, O'Grady & Elkin, 1992).

Intervention Fidelity as a Mediator of Outcome. In most psychotherapy outcome studies, fidelity is reported as a simple average or range of compliance, to confirm that the therapy has been implemented consistently (e.g., Clarke, Hawkins, Murphy, Sheeber, Lewinsohn & Seeley, 1995). In efficacy trials, where the main effects of the intervention are the primary concern, the aim is to maximize program fidelity, assuming that this will lead to the best outcomes. Beyond this simple confirmation of protocol compliance, however, these ratings may be examined as a possible mediator of outcome. Only a few mental health treatment studies have examined this issue, and most of these have been in the adult psychotherapy outcome literature where the relationship between therapy adherence and outcome in these studies has been mixed (e.g., Barber, Crits-Christoph & Luborsky, 1996; DeRubeis & Feeley, 1990).

In one of the few child psychotherapy adherence investigations, Henggeler, Melton, Brondino, Scherer and Hanley (1996) found that chronic juvenile offender outcomes were substantially better in Multisystemic Therapy when treatment adherence ratings were high. In contrast to the child treatment literature, Durlak (in this volume) identifies numerous prevention trials in which higher program adherence has been associated with better outcomes.

The remainder of this paper reviews intervention adherence in four adolescent depression randomized outcome trials conducted by our research team: two treatment studies (Lewinsohn, Clarke, Hops & Andrews, 1990; Lewinsohn, Clarke, Rohde, Hops & Seeley, 1996), one primary prevention trial (Clarke, Hawkins, Murphy & Sheeber, 1991) and a targeted prevention trial (Clarke, Hawkins, Murphy, Sheeber, Lewinsohn & Seeley, 1995). All four outcome trials share several common theoretical, intervention, assessment and fidelity methodological elements, reviewed below.

Theoretical Background. Our prevention and treatment programs are based on the multifactorial model of depression (Lewinsohn, Hoberman, Teri & Hautzinger, 1985), in which depression results from multiple etiological elements acting either alone or in combination, including negative cognitions, stressful events, predisposing vulnerabilities/risk factors (e.g., being female, having depressed parents) and immunities to depression (e.g., high self-esteem, coping skills). Teaching individuals new coping techniques and strategies provides them with some "immunity" against the development of depressive disorders (or a means of terminating a current episode).

Interventions. Central to the issue of intervention fidelity is the use of manualized cognitive-behavioral interventions in all studies. Treatment and prevention intervention manuals and adolescent workbooks were highly structured, with explicit scripts and prescribed activities for each session. The group intervention employed in the two *treatment* studies was the Adolescent Coping With Depression Course (CWDA; Clarke, Lewinsohn & Hops, 1990), typically delivered by a single therapist to a mixed-gender group of six to ten adolescents (ages 14 to 18) in 16 two-hour sessions, twice a week for eight weeks. Sessions provide skills training to help control depressed mood: changing irrational/negative thinking, increasing pleasant activities, reducing anxiety through relaxation training, social skills training, reducing conflict and negotiating solutions to common family problems, life planning and goal setting and depression relapse prevention. The CWDA program is a modification of the original adult Coping With Depression Course (Lewinsohn, Antonuccio, Steinmetz & Teri, 1984), with simplified exercises and instructions, more role-play and less didactic materials, and illustrative cartoons in the workbook.

The targeted prevention study (Clarke et al., 1995) employed a shorter version of the CWDA Course, limited to fifteen 45-minute sessions to facilitate delivery at schools after regular classes. This program, called the Coping with Stress class (CWS; Clarke & Lewinsohn, 1995), focused on depression prevention through controlling irrational and negative thinking patterns (only one component of the CWDA treatment program). The CWS course targeted youth whose subdiagnostic depressive symptomatology was insufficient to meet full DSM affective disorder criteria, but who have an increased risk for subsequent full episodes of depression (Weissman, Myers, Thompson & Belanger, 1986). Our rationale for focusing exclusively on the cognitive restructuring skills training in the prevention program was partly pragmatic, dictated by the need to shorten the overall program. However, the choice of cognitive therapy over the other components in the full CWDA treatment program (relaxation therapy, increasing pleasant activities, conflict reduction) was justified by studies supporting this domain as a specific risk factor for future depression (Hammen, 1988; Jaenicke, Hammen, Zupan, Hiroto, Gordon, Adrian and Burge, 1987). Two other research groups (e.g., Beardslee et al., 1993; Jaycox, Reivich, Gillham & Seligman, 1994) have employed similar cognitive therapy approaches to prevent depressive disorder and/or symptoms in at-risk youth, providing some post-hoc support for this choice.

The primary prevention program consisted of five 45-minute sessions taught in high school health classes by teachers, with the goal of preventing depressive mood in an unselected (normal) population. Adolescents were taught to increase their rate of pleasant activities, using an abbreviated version of the pleasant activities section of the CWDA treatment program (Clarke et al., 1990), reworked for a non-depressed population. The behavioral skills were selected rather than another intervention modality (e.g., cognitive therapy skills) because it is the easiest to teach in a brief intervention, and was most likely to be acceptable to the many non-depressed youth in the target audience.

Therapists for the targeted prevention and treatment programs were provided with 40 to 60 hours of intervention training. However, health class teachers were provided only two hours of training to deliver the primary prevention program. Training included a supervised mock group consisting of other adult trainees playing the role of adolescents. The supervisor stopped at appropriate points to provide feedback or describe typical group process issues. Additional supervision was provided periodically during ongoing trials to address clinical issues that arose (e.g., suicidal youth), and to encourage continuing compliance with the treatment protocol (to minimize "drift" over time).

Assessment. Each study employed similar assessment methodology, except as noted. Depression and other psychiatric diagnoses were assessed in both the treatment studies and the targeted prevention trial by a semi-structured psychiatric interview, the Children's Schedule for Affective Disorders and Schizophrenia (K-SADS; Orvaschel & Puig-Antich, 1986). Depression symptomatology was also assessed in all four studies for principal outcome analyses, using either the Beck Depression Inventory (Beck et al., 1961) or the Center for Epidemiological Studies–Depression Scale (Ratloff, 1977). A variety of other measures of mediating and moderating variables were also employed (Andrews, Lewinsohn, Hops & Roberts, 1993).

Fidelity Methodology. Most pertinent to this report is the measurement of intervention fidelity. All intervention sessions in all four studies were audio or video-taped, barring infrequent equipment failure. For the two treatment trials and the targeted prevention study, recordings of three sessions were randomly selected from each group for fidelity review by a senior supervisor. Almost all sessions of the primary prevention program were observed by a live research assistant who made ratings using the fidelity scale.

Fidelity Scale. Each recorded or observed session was rated on a 10-item fidelity scale. Each item was rated on a three-point scale: either No Adherence (0), Partial Adherence (1) or Complete Adherence (2), yielding a total compliance score of 0 to 12 for each session, and a range of 0 to 36 for the total of all three reviewed sessions per intervention group. The first four scale items address protocol compliance: Did the therapist review previous session material via oral review questions and/or a review of homework? Did the therapist provide structured practice for skills and techniques during session? Did the therapist deliver the entire lecture as outlined in the leader manual? Did the therapist clearly assign homework? The latter five scale items address intervention process issues. These include: What was the overall tone of the session (up, neutral or down)? Did the therapist attempt to provide approximately equal speaking time for all members? Did the therapist express ideas clearly and at an appropriate pace? Was the therapist organized? Did the therapist keep class members on task during session? The final item (How difficult was the group to work with in this session?) is separate from either subscale.

The fidelity scale was modified by Peter Lewinsohn for the first of the CWDA treatment trials, starting with items from several other protocol compliance scales, developed earlier for use in adult psychotherapy outcome trials (Baffa & Steinmetz, 1982; DeRubeis, Hollon, Evans & Bemis, 1982; Hollon, Elkin-Waskow, Evans, & Lowrey, 1984; Young & Beck, 1980).

As mentioned, all intervention sessions were either observed or recorded using audio or videotape. Because therapists did not know which sessions would be reviewed, they were potentially observable for the entire intervention and presumably motivated to follow the protocol closely for all sessions. In addition, fidelity ratings were used in supervision sessions to provide feedback to therapists to help shape better "on-task" behavior. High fidelity was also enhanced by the detailed nature of the intervention manuals, which provided scripted dialog for many of the sections. Although therapists were free to use their own words, they were asked to retain the key concepts in every section. This had the effect of allowing little opportunity for therapists to deviate from the main lectures and exercises. These restrictions sometimes frustrated therapists, but they had the effect of yielding high fidelity. While we cannot say whether our programs were too structured and restrictive, and whether there is an ideal level of manual detail, these issues could be tested in properly designed studies (Clarke, 1995).

Psychometric Properties of the Fidelity Measure. In the first treatment study, at least one of the three tapes reviewed for each group was re-rated by a different rater in order to calculate inter-rater reliability. The average Kappa across the 14 reliability sessions was .69 (SD = .10; range = .51 to .81), indicating good reliability. Inter-rated reliability data was not available for the second treatment study.

In the first treatment study, Cronbach's alpha was .72 for all scale items (.57 for the compliance subscale, and .56 for the therapy process subscale). In the second treatment study, overall Cronbach's alpha was .57 for all scale items (compliance and process subscale alphas were .38 and .60, respectively). These relatively low-to-moderate alpha scores are somewhat lower than reported for other therapy adherence rating scales (e.g., Barber & Crits-Christoph, 1996), and may be due to several factors. First, the total scale consists of only 10 items; fewer items generally limits the upper bounds of the internal consistency of a scale (this is even more relevant for the two subscales). Second, we generally had good compliance, with little variability in scores. Thus, low compliance in one area may not be that predictive of low compliance in another area, which also limits internal consistency. Paradoxically, if we had poorer overall compliance (e.g., greater variability), we might have found better scale reliability.

Treatment Studies 1 and 2. We conducted two group CBT treatment trials with actively depressed youth, the first study from 1986 to 1988 (with a sample of 59 youth; Lewinsohn et al., 1990) and the second study from 1989 to 1993 (with a sample of 96 youth; Lewinsohn et al., 1996). In both studies, adolescents with current unipolar depressive disorder were randomly assigned to one of three conditions: (a) only adolescents enrolled in the group CBT program, (b) adolescents enrolled in the group CBT with parent(s) enrolled in a separate parent group, or (c) a wait-list control condition. In both studies, active treatments resulted in significantly greater subject improvement relative to the control condition. However, no consistent difference was detected between the two active conditions, suggesting no incremental advantage for parent involvement. Follow-up of the two treatment conditions suggested reasonable persistence of effects, with depression relapse rates ranging from 20% to 25% by two years post-treatment, lower than reported for treated depressed adults (Belsher & Costello, 1988).

Intervention fidelity ratings for the active treatments in both studies indicated high and consistent implementation of the CBT program (Table 1). Fidelity ranged from 44% to 100% in the first study, while in the second it ranged from 67% to 100%. This suggests some tightening of the variability in fidelity over time, although this could have easily been due to changes in therapist staff over that time. In both cases, however, the moderately high fidelity ratings (particularly in the second trial) truncated the range over which we could observe the relationship between fidelity variation and treatment outcome.

Primary Prevention Study. Intervention fidelity data was collected for only one of two primary prevention trials we conducted in 1990 (Clarke, Hawkins, Murphy & Sheeber, 1991). In this trial, seven high school health classrooms (with 190 total subjects) were randomized to a five-session prevention condition, while seven classes also with 190 subjects were randomized to the "usual curriculum" control condition. None of the subjects in this universal prevention trial were selected as having any elevated risk of depression. Subjects were assessed with the CES-D at the first and final sessions, and at a 12-week follow-up. Unfortunately, no persistent program effects were noted for boys, girls, or extreme scoring cases. These negative findings may have been the result of an inactive intervention, a too-small sample, and/or subjects who failed to use the

TABLE 1. Intervention Fidelity Scores for Four Adolescent Depression Treatment and Prevention Studies

		Compliance Scores		
Study Type	No. Rated Sessions	Mean	(SD)	Range
Treatment 1 (Lewinsohn et al., 1990)	14 groups × 3 sessions each = 42 rated sessions	77.5%	(9.5)	44.4%-100%
Treatment 2 (Lewinsohn et al., 1996)	24 groups × 3 sessions each = 72 rated sessions	90.5%	(9.0)	66.7%-100%
Primary Prevention (Clarke et al., 1991)	7 groups × 5 sessions each = 34 rated sessions[a]	86.2%	(8.4)	61.1%-100%
Targeted Prevention (Clarke et al., 1995)	7 groups × 3 sessions each = 21 rated sessions	93.9%	(5.2)	77.8%-100%

[a] Fidelity ratings were not made for one session of the 35 possible sessions.

behavioral skills and therefore received no benefit. An additional explanation for the poor results was possible inadequate implementation of the program by health class teachers. However, the collection of intervention fidelity ratings allowed us to rule this out with some confidence. As seen in Table 1, teacher compliance with the protocol ranged from 61% to 100% compliance, suggesting that teachers followed the detailed manual to a satisfactory degree.

Targeted Prevention Study. The purpose of this trial was to reduce the incidence of unipolar affective disorders and symptomatology in high-school adolescents at risk for future depression (Clarke et al., 1995). Ninth-grade adolescents with an elevated risk for depression were identified in two stages: (a) a school-wide administration of the CES-D to 1,640 adolescents in 9th grade health classes; and (b) a subsequent confirmatory structured diagnostic interview (the K-SADS) for the 222 consenting adolescents with a CES-D cutoff score of 24 or greater. Subjects with current affective diagnoses (n = 47) were referred to non-study services, and 25 adolescents either declined to participate further or were excluded for problem behavior. The remaining 150 adolescents, not currently depressed but with elevated CES-D scores, were randomly assigned to (a) the CWS preventive intervention described earlier (n = 74); or (b) a "usual care" control condition (n = 76). Survival analysis results indicate significantly less cumulative MDD and/or dysthymia in the experimental group (14.5%) at a median 13-month follow-up relative to the control group (25.7%).

As with the two treatment studies, protocol adherence ratings for the prevention program were high, ranging from 78% to 100% (Table 1). These ratings were particularly gratifying, as this study was much more of an effectiveness trial than the two treatment outcome studies. Prevention therapists were unpaid school counselors who volunteered to implement the program. While we provided extensive training and ongoing supervision, school counselors were not directly answerable to the research project, unlike our treatment study therapists (who were employees). There are at least two reasons why school counselors may have adhered to the protocol as well as they did. First, structured protocols are much more common in the school setting (e.g., instructional curricula) than in general psychosocial treatment settings. School counselors often taught academic subjects and may have been more comfortable with following the structured protocol, especially compared to a mental health therapist not affiliated with schools. Second, we believe that interventionists just learning a new approach may be more comfortable with (and may even appreciate) structured psycho-educational or teaching materials (Hibbs et al., in press). This includes many "cross over" professionals (e.g., health teachers, school counselors, primary health care providers) who do not regularly deliver behavioral health interventions and may appreciate a level of guidance which might be perceived as too restrictive by full-time mental health specialists.

Difficulties Examining the Association Between Fidelity and Outcome. Although evaluation of the mediating effects of program fidelity in child and adolescent mental health studies is desirable, several aspects of our particular methodology complicate a reasonable test of this question in our four studies. Perhaps most prohibitive is the fact that our CBT programs are delivered in a group or class format, with six to 10 youth per group (and 30 youth in the primary prevention program). The "unit of analysis" issue (Hopkins, 1982) significantly hampers our ability to detect mediating effects of fidelity in these circumstances. For example, our targeted prevention study (Clarke et al., 1995) had an active intervention sample of 74 youth enrolled, or "nested," in 7 groups. Fidelity ratings were made for therapists serving an entire group, not an individual youth. Thus, for fidelity analyses we have a sample of seven groups, some of which were led by the same school counselor in sequential cohorts (necessitating another level of nesting and further complicating the sample issue). Clearly this is too small a sample to be confident of detecting anything but an enormously large fidelity mediating effect. Although fidelity ratings were made for three separate sessions from each group, these cannot be considered independent observations since fidelity ratings for any three sessions for the same therapist leading the same group are likely to be highly inter-correlated. This has the net effect of making it very difficult to detect an association between *group* intervention fidelity and mean group member improvement.

Another limitation, if it can be called that, is that we worked very diligently to maximize intervention fidelity in these studies, based on the assumption that this would yield the best outcomes. Ongoing supervision and feedback were provided to group leaders in order to improve fidelity and reduce drift away from the protocol over time. While this is desirable in efficacy outcome trials, these circumstances are not the best for detecting an effect of fidelity on outcome (see Henggeler et al., 1996). The low variability in adherence ratings, and the positively skewed distribution (e.g., a "ceiling" effect) again conspire against detecting any but the largest mediating effects.

What, if anything, would facilitate analysis of the mediating effects of intervention fidelity? If retaining a group intervention in future studies, we continue to be limited to fidelity ratings for the much smaller sample of groups rather than for individuals. One solution is to switch to individual therapy, with separate protocol adherence ratings unique to each therapist-client pair. However, what if we wish to remain with a group modality? One intermediate solution would be to obtain "subject-specific" fidelity ratings: that is, how well did the therapist implement the session for each participant? Several shortcomings of this approach are immediately evident. While some group members are more successfully engaged by the therapist in a given session than other group members, this is probably not consistently observable. There are many group activities (role plays, discussions, modeling) which often benefit the entire membership but which may not be captured by ratings of interactions between therapists and individual group members. Another possibility is to have subjects make ratings of fidelity from their own perspective. This, however, requires patients to recognize on-task therapist behavior when they see it, or at least to judge how well a group leader followed a pre-defined assessment protocol. This would seem as difficult a task as therapy itself. While general patient satisfaction ratings are available, these do not wholly capture the fidelity construct but may be confounded with other process factors (similarity to therapist, attraction, degree of improvement). Overall, this seems an unresolved issue.

Regarding the high mean fidelity rating scores and positively skewed distribution in our studies, the main solution appears to be a methodological transition from efficacy to effectiveness trials. In the former (including most of our studies), intervention fidelity is pushed to the maximum through various incentives, supervision and checks (such as videotaping). In effectiveness trials, intervention implementation is often more naturalistic and consistent with usual care. For example, an ideal circumstance for testing the fidelity-outcome relationship would be to permit therapists to implement the groups with minimal guidelines (other than the manual) and no penalties for deviation from the protocol. This would likely result in a more normal distribution of protocol adherence, with a mean fidelity rating closer to 50% compliance (or at least lower than the mean in efficacy trials). Interestingly, these are similar to the circumstances found in the one child psychotherapy study (Henggeler et al., 1996) that found an association between protocol adherence and outcome.

Conclusions. The results of the Henggeler et al. (1996) study and the substance abuse prevention trials reviewed by Durlak (this volume) have substantial implications. First, outcome trials of mental health treatment and prevention programs should measure and report basic intervention fidelity, and, whenever possible, examine the mediating effects of adherence on outcome. Second, greater thought should be given to whether or not supervision efforts should be designed to maximize protocol adherence (as in typical efficacy trials) or to permit protocol adherence to vary naturally (as in typical effectiveness trials), or whether to conduct a controlled hybrid trial of these two extremes (as suggested in Clarke, 1995). Finally, although it is premature to conclude that fidelity is the primary key to maximizing intervention success, non-research clinical practitioners and prevention specialists may wish to re-examine their implementation for fidelity to original protocols in light of the limited data available so far (see Weisz, Donenberg, Han & Weiss, 1995). At the very least, practitioners and policy makers need to be aware of the issues and emerging views on treatment and prevention adherence, to be prepared to act quickly when more compelling and confirming data are available.

Are there situations where maximizing protocol adherence may be counter-productive? It is not that difficult to imagine situations where a slavish persistence in a protocol is ineffective, or worse, harmful. Persistence in Behavior A when Behavior B is called for may even lead to poorer outcome. High fidelity to a rigorous protocol which doesn't allow much deviation to "fit" the situation may not be desirable, particularly for conditions which have serious and acute associated problems or manifestations (e.g., suicide attempts in depressed youth, or drug overdoses in substance abusing teens).

Another situation which requires careful forethought about protocol adherence is the recent emergence of pre-defined but flexible protocols, guided by "if-then" algorithms (see Jensen, Hibbs & Pilkonis, 1996). For example, the protocol for the Mutlimodal Treatment Study for Children with ADHD (MTA; Hinshaw, 1996) permits switching and tailoring treatments to meet the family and youth's needs according to a hierarchical decision-making tree. Is it possible to assess fidelity for this type of protocol? Such judgements would be more difficult, and would likely involve more clinical judgements on the part of the rater (and thus more opportunity for error in assessing fidelity).

Finally, assessment of intervention fidelity should distinguish between fidelity to the program versus competence in the delivery of the program. Two interventionists may have identical adherence ratings, but may differ substantially in their insightful use of techniques, the appropriateness of their responses to clinical presentations of subjects, and in a word, competency. Research in adult psychotherapy outcome suggests that adherence and competence, while related, may have somewhat independent relationships with intervention outcome (see Barber, Crits-Christoph, & Luborsky, 1996; Luborsky & Barber, 1993). Only when the complex relationship between these three constructs is well understood will we be fully armed to train and supervise program delivery staff to maximize intervention outcomes.

REFERENCES

Andrews, J.A., Lewinsohn, P.M., Hops, H. & Roberts, R.E. (1993). Psychometric properties of scales for the measurement of psychosocial variables associated with depression in adolescence. *Psychological Reports, 73*, 1019-1046.

Baffa, G.A. & Steinmetz, J. (1982). *Behavior therapy scale rating manual.* Unpublished manuscript, Center for the Study of Psychotherapy and Aging, Palo Alto, CA.

Barber, J.P. & Crits-Christoph, P. (1996). Development of a therapist adherence/competence rating scale for supportive-expressive dynamic psychotherapy: A preliminary report. *Psychotherapy Research, 6*, 81-94.

Barber, J.P., Crits-Christoph, P. & Luborsky, L. (1996). Effects of therapist adherence and competence on patient outcome in brief dynamic therapy. *Journal of Consulting and Clinical Psychology, 64*, 619-622.

Beardslee, W.R., Salt, P., Porterfield, K., Rothberg, P.C., van de Velde, P., Swatling, S., Hoke, L., Moilanen, D.L., Wheelock, I. (1993). Comparison of preventive interventions for families with parental affective disorder. *Journal of the American Academy of Child and Adolescent Psychiatry, 32*, 254-263.

Beck, A. T., Rush, A. J., Shaw, B. F., & Emery, G. (1979). *Cognitive therapy of depression*. New York: Guilford.

Beck, A. T., Ward, C. H., Mendelson, M., Mock, J. E., & Erbaugh, J. K. (1961). An inventory for measuring depression. *Archives of General Psychiatry, 4*, 561-571.

Belsher, G. & Costello, C.G. (1988). Relapse after recovery from unipolar depression: A critical review. *Psychological Bulletin, 104*, 84-96.

Clarke, G.N. (1995). Improving the transition from basic efficacy research to effectiveness studies: Methodological issues and procedures. *Journal of Consulting and Clinical Psychology, 63*, 718-725.

Clarke, G.N., Hawkins, W., Murphy, M., & Sheeber, L. (1993). School-based primary prevention of depressive symptomatology in adolescents: Findings from two studies. *Journal of Adolescent Research, 8*, 183-204.

Clarke, G.N., Hawkins, W., Murphy, M., Sheeber, L., Lewinsohn, P.M., & Seeley, J.R. (1995). Targeted prevention of unipolar depressive disorder in an at-risk sample of high school adolescents: A randomized trial of a group cognitive intervention. *Journal of the American Academy of Child and Adolescent Psychiatry, 34*, 312-321.

Clarke, G.N., Lewinsohn, P.M., & Hops, H. (1990). *Instructor's manual for the Adolescent Coping with Depression Course*. Eugene, Oregon: Castalia Press.

DeRubeis, R. & Feeley, M. (1990). Determinants of change in cognitive therapy for depression. *Cognitive Therapy and Research, 14*, 469-482.

DeRubeis, R.J., Hollon, S.D., Evans, M.D. & Bemis, K.M. (1982). Can psychotherapies for depression be discriminated? A systematic investigation of cognitive therapy and interpersonal therapy. *Journal of Consulting and Clinical Psychology, 50*, 744-756.

Durlak, J.A. (1998). Why program implementation is important. *Journal of Prevention & Intervention in the Community, 17(2).*

Hammen, C. (1988). Self-cognitions, stressful events, and the prediction of depression in children of depressed mothers. *Journal of Abnormal Child Psychology, 16*, 347-360.

Henggeler, S.W., Melton, G.B., Brondino, M.J. Scherer, D.G. & Hanley, J.H. (1996). *Multisystemic therapy with violent and chronic offenders and their families: The role of treatment fidelity in successful dissemination*. Presented at a meeting of the NIMH Child Services Research Branch, Bethesda, MD.

Henggeler, S.W. Melton, G.B. & Smith, L.A. (1992). Family preservation using Multisystemic Therapy: An effective alternative to incarcerating serious juvenile offenders. *Journal of Consulting and Clinical Psychology, 60*, 953-961.

Hibbs, E.D., Clarke, G.N., Hechtman, L., Abikoff, H.B., Greenhill, L.L. & Jensen, P.S. (in press). Manual development for the treatment of child and adolescent disorders. *Psychopharmacology Bulletin*.

Hibbs, E.D. & Jensen, P.S. (1996). *Psychosocial treatments for children and adolescent disorders: Empirically based strategies for clinical practice.* Washington, D.C.: American Psychiatric Assoc. Press.

Hill, C.E., O'Grady, K.E. & Elkin, I. (1992). Applying the Collaborative Study Psychotherapy Rating Scale to rate therapist adherence in cognitive-behavior therapy, interpersonal therapy, and clinical management. *Journal of Consulting and Clinical Psychology, 60,* 73-79.

Hinshaw, S.P. (1996). Enhancing social competence: Integrating self-management strategies with behavioral procedures for children with ADHD. In E.D. Hibbs & P.S. Jensen (Eds.), *Psychosocial treatments for children and adolescent disorders: Empirically based strategies for clinical practice* (pp. 285-310). Washington, D.C.: American Psychiatric Assoc. Press.

Hollon, S.D., Elkin-Waskow, I., Evans, M. & Lowrey, H.A. (1984). *System for rating therapies for depression.* Paper presented at the annual meeting of the American Psychological Association.

Hopkins, K.D. (1982). The unit of analysis: Group means versus individual observations. *American Educational Research Journal, 19,* 5-18.

Jacobson, N.S., Dobson, K.S., Truax, P.A., Addis, M.E., Koerner, K., Gollan, J.K., Gortner, E. & Prince, S.E. (1996). A component analysis of cognitive-behavioral treatment for depression. *Journal of Consulting and Clinical Psychology, 64,* 295-304.

Jaenicke, C., Hammen, C., Zupan, B., Hiroto, D., Gordon, D., Adrian, C., & Burge, D. (1987). Cognitive vulnerability in children at risk for depression. *Journal of Abnormal Child Psychology, 15,* 559-572.

Jaycox, L.H., Reivich, K.J., Gillham, J. & Seligman, M.E. (1994). Prevention of depressive symptoms in school children. *Behaviour Research & Therapy, 32,* 801-816.

Jensen, P.S., Hibbs, E.D. & Pilkonis, P.A. (1996). From ivory tower to clinical practice: Future directions for child and adolescent psychotherapy research. In E.D. Hibbs & P.S. Jensen (Eds.), *Psychosocial treatments for children and adolescent disorders: Empirically based strategies for clinical practice* (pp. 701-712). Washington, D.C.: American Psychiatric Assoc. Press.

Lambert, M.J., Garfield, D.A. & Bergin, A.E. (1986). The effectiveness of psychotherapy. In S.L. Garfield & A.E. Bergin (Eds.), *Handbook of psychotherapy and behavior change* (pp. 157-212). New York: Wiley & Sons.

Lewinsohn, P.M., Antonuccio, D.O., Steinmetz, J., & Teri, L. (1984). *The coping with depression course: A psychoeducational intervention for unipolar depression.* Eugene, OR: Castalia Press.

Lewinsohn, P.M., Clarke, G.N., Hops, H., & Andrews, J. (1990). Cognitive-behavioral group treatment of depression in adolescents. *Behavior Therapy, 21,* 385-401.

Lewinsohn, P.M., Clarke, G.N., Rohde, P., Hops, H., & Seeley, J.R. (1996). A course in coping: A cognitive-behavioral approach to the treatment of adolescent depression. In E.D. Hibbs & P.S. Jensen (Eds.), *Psychosocial treatments for children and adolescent disorders: Empirically based strategies for clinical practice* (pp. 109-135). Washington, D.C.: American Psychiatric Assoc. Press.

Lewinsohn, P.M., Hoberman, H.M., Teri, L., & Hautzinger, M. (1985). An integrative theory of unipolar depression. In S. Reiss, and R.R. Bootzin (Eds.), *Theoretical issues in behavioral therapy* (pp. 313-359). New York: Academic Press.

Luborsky, L. & Barber, J.P. (1993). Benefits of adherence to treatment manuals, and where to get them. In N. Miller, L. Luborsky, J.P. Barber & J.P. Docherty (Eds.), *Psychodynamic treatment research: A handbook for clinical practice* (pp. 211-226). New York: Basic Books.

Orvaschel, H., & Puig-Antich, J. (1986). *Schedule for affective disorder and schizophrenia for school-age children. Epidemiologic version: Kiddie-SADS-E (K-SADS-E) (4th version).* Technical report, Western Psychiatric Institute and Clinic, Pittsburgh, PA.

Radloff, L. S. (1977). A CES-D scale: A self-report depression scale for research in the general population. *Applied Psychological Measurement, 1*, 385-401.

Weissman, M.W., Myers, J.K., Thompson, W.C. & Belanger, A. (1986). Depressive symptoms as a risk factor for major depression. In Erlenmeyer-Kimling, L., Miller, N.E. (Eds.), *Life-span research on the prediction of psychopathology* (pp. 251-260). Hillsdale, NJ: Erlbaum.

Weisz, J.R., Donenberg, G.R., Han, S.S. & Weiss, B. (1995). Bridging the gap between laboratory and clinic in child and adolescent psychotherapy. *Journal of Consulting and Clinical Psychology, 63*, 688-701.

Young, J. & Beck, A.T. (1980). *Cognitive therapy scale rating manual.* Unpublished manuscript, Center for Cognitive Therapy, Philadelphia, PA.

Zeiss, A., Lewinsohn, P.M., & Munoz, R.F. (1979). Nonspecific improvement effects in depression using interpersonal skills training, pleasant activity schedules, or cognitive training. *Journal of Consulting and Clinical Psychology, 47*, 427-439.

Zimmerman, J.K., Asnis, G.M., & Schwartz, B.J. (1995). Enhancing outpatient treatment compliance: A multifamily psychoeducational intake group. In J. K. Zimmerman & G.M. Asnis (Eds.), *Treatment approaches with suicidal adolescents* (pp. 106-134). New York, NY: John Wiley & Sons.

Implementing a Violence Intervention for Inner-City Adolescents: Potential Pitfalls and Suggested Remedies

Paulette Moore Hines
Cathaleene Macias
Tatiana Perrino

University of Medicine and Dentistry of New Jersey

SUMMARY. Violence is a growing public health problem that disproportionately affects African American adolescents. There is a pressing need for more attention to be directed to the development of theoretically-based, research-validated, culturally sensitive preventive interventions and programs. This article focuses on the steps involved in the development, implementation, and evaluation of a culturally-specific program designed to reduce the prevalence of violent behaviors and related injuries and deaths among urban, African American teens. The project's success was heavily dependent upon the commitment and cooperation of the community organizations that participated in the field research. Although numerous unexpected challenges were encountered, the preliminary findings indi-

Address correspondence to: Paulette Hines, University of Medicine and Dentistry of New Jersey, Office of Prevention Services, P.O. Box 1392, Piscataway, NJ 08855-1392.

This research was supported by the State of New Jersey Department of Health and Senior Services, Division of Family Health Services Grant # 97-158-IPC-00 awarded to the first author.

[Haworth co-indexing entry note]: "Implementing a Violence Intervention for Inner-City Adolescents: Potential Pitfalls and Suggested Remedies." Hines, Paulette Moore, Cathaleene Macias, and Tatiana Perrino. Co-published simultaneously in *Journal of Prevention & Intervention in the Community* (The Haworth Press, Inc.) Vol. 17, No. 2, 1998, pp. 35-49; and: *Program Implementation in Preventive Trials* (ed: Joseph A. Durlak, and Joseph R. Ferrari) The Haworth Press, Inc., 1998, pp. 35-49. Single or multiple copies of this article are available for a fee from The Haworth Document Delivery Service [1-800-342-9678, 9:00 a.m. - 5:00 p.m. (EST). E-mail address: getinfo@haworthpressinc.com].

cate that it is possible to effectively implement preventive interventions in urban communities with modest funding. *[Article copies available for a fee from The Haworth Document Delivery Service: 1-800-342-9678. E-mail address: getinfo@haworth.com]*

Violence is a major public health problem that threatens the health and lives of America's next generation of adults, particularly African American males and those living in poverty (Christoffel, 1990). Homicide is the 12th leading cause of death in the United States over all (rate of 10.6 per 100,000), the second leading cause of death for 15 to 24 year-olds, and the leading cause of death for African American males and females in that age group (National Center for Injury Prevention and Control, 1995).

In spite of the gravity of these facts, the study of the prevention of antisocial behavior is very much in its infancy and has been the focus of relatively few empirical studies (Kazdin, 1991) (O'Donnell, Cohen & Hausman, 1990). Even fewer have documented the issues involved in translating models for preventive intervention into real world applications (Powell & Hawkins, 1996). This paper focuses on the steps involved in the initial development and field testing of SANKOFA, a culturally-specific program designed to reduce the prevalence of violent behaviors and related injuries and deaths among urban, African American adolescents. Although SANKOFA is a multi-level (i.e., adolescents, parents, service providers), multi-component intervention (i.e., skills training and case management), this paper will focus on the adolescent skills training component.

EVALUATION DESIGN AND METHODS

The major aims of the project have been: (1) to determine the overall effectiveness of the SANKOFA intervention for reducing youth violence, youth victimization by violence, and youth participation in behaviors precipitating violence; and (2) to evaluate the differential effectiveness of SANKOFA for specific subgroups of adolescents, including youth with differing levels of familial support, youth in mainstream public high schools, youth with classified behavioral problems, youth who have dropped out of school, and youth who have self-reported problems with impulse control.

The ongoing SANKOFA research project has a quasi-experimental, repeated measure research design. Subjects were randomly assigned to one of two conditions: (1) a violence prevention training group; or (2) a no intervention comparison group. Measures were selected or developed with consideration of the developmental and cultural characteristics of the target population, psychometric properties and feedback from colleagues in the field. Current pre and post research measures for the adolescent intervention include a violence survey and a questionnaire designed to assess changes in participants' knowledge, attitudes, and behavioral intentions.

IMPLEMENTATION STEPS AND CHALLENGES

The implementation of the SANKOFA research study involved numerous interrelated, overlapping levels of action. A description of 12 key implementation steps, the expected and unanticipated difficulties encountered during implementation, and the actions taken to address these implementation issues follow.

1. Conduct Focus Groups/Meet with Key Informants

Preventive interventions are likely to be most effective when targeted for the intended audience. Project SANKOFA staff met with adolescents from the organizations that were intended to be research sites. We solicited the youths' perceptions regarding violence in their community (e.g., reasons teens fight, types of weapons used, typical scenarios) as well as their suggestions regarding sites for implementation, and incentives for participation, etc. In addition, meetings were held with parents and youth service providers to secure their ideas on the proposed implementation plan.

2. Formulate a Theoretical Framework

Efforts to develop effective violence prevention interventions are likely to be most successful if they are based on a solid theoretical foundation. After careful review of the literature, a decision was reached to utilize the theory of planned behavior (Ajzen, 1991; Madden, Ellen, & Ajzen, 1992) as the framework to guide our intervention. According to the theory of planned behavior, behavior is determined by specific behavioral intentions, which in turn, are determined by both attitudes toward the specific behavior and subjective norms regarding the behavior. In other words, people intend to perform a behavior (e.g., fighting) when they evaluate that behavior positively and when they believe significant others (e.g., peers, parents) think they should perform it.

The theory of planned behavior has affinity with the social cognitive theory construct of perceived self-efficacy (Bandura, 1989). If people believe that they have little control over performing a behavior because of a lack of requisite skills or resources, their intentions to perform the behavior may be low even if they have favorable attitudes or supportive subjective norms regarding it. The suggestion, therefore, is that if adolescents lack necessary skills, their intentions to respond violently to a provocation may be increased. They may believe that they have no other option but to respond violently even if they have nonviolent attitudes and they perceive normative support for nonviolence (Ajzen and Madden, 1986). In turn, variables that are external to the model (e.g., ethnic identity) should affect specific behavioral intentions and behaviors by influencing attitudes toward those behaviors, subjective norms regarding them, and perceptions of control over them (Ajzen 1991; Fishbein & Middlestadt, 1989).

3. Develop the Adolescent Curriculum

Formulation of the adolescent curriculum began with a review of the literature to identify constructs previously determined or proposed to be relevant to the aims of the SANKOFA intervention and to determine the relative effectiveness of various training methods and other issues that might impact implementation. Information secured from focus groups with the teens was used to inform the mini-lectures and to help formulate relevant scenarios for case analyses and role plays. Key issues that required consideration included: content (i.e., What information and skills should be given priority?), ordering (i.e., What sequence will maximize development of the desired cognitive and behavioral skills?), and time (i.e., What amount of time should be devoted to each topic? How much emphasis should be placed on cognitive vs. behavioral skills? How lengthy should the program be in order to accomplish the training objectives but not jeopardize its adoption and support by different schools and organizations?) Additional concerns included: the organization of the curriculum components into discrete, one-hour teaching modules that address a measurable construct, role play construction, and the formulation of the curriculum to maximize the extent to which it is engaging, responsive to different learning styles, and minimizes boredom. A variety of active training strategies are used throughout the curriculum. The strategies employed include brief, didactic presentations, games, self-directed learning, interactive exercises, group discussions, brainstorming, visuals, videos, modeling, role playing, and behavioral rehearsal.

The aforementioned process led to the development of a two phase curriculum: an initial intervention comprised of 24 one-hour modules and booster training 3 months later which consists of three one-hour modules.

The project name, SANKOFA–a term of African origin–was selected because the meaning "reaching back to our past in order to move forward" is consistent with the premises underpinning the curriculum and the emphasis placed on cultural heritage.

A number of strategies were employed to maximize the cultural sensitivity of the curriculum. Each session begins and ends with a talking circle, a group process in which the value of everyone's voice being heard is symbolized by the passing of an object of cultural significance (an ankh) as each group member speaks. Proverbs of African and African American origin are introduced and discussed at the beginning of each module to help participants focus on the theme of the module. Video segments from popular movies are used to introduce and/or elaborate on various topics. Teaching fables from African tradition, program values that draw from African American tradition, a program motto, and an emphasis on topics (e.g., internalized racism) of high relevance to urban, minority youth are additional means of increasing the cultural familiarity, credibility, and relevance of the material that is taught.

4. Solicit/Sustain Community Support

During the project planning phase, an advisory group was formed of representatives from the organizations selected to be research sites as well as from other community organizations, local government, and religious institutions. The advisory group evaluated the implementation plan; they offered recommendations regarding unanticipated implementation challenges (e.g., the need to replace research sites), strategies to promote community support, and supplemental funding sources. Advisory group members also actively participated in disseminating information about the project and informing staff about environment shifts that might impact the project.

As anticipated, SANKOFA staff faced some suspiciousness regarding the research project. Individual meetings were held with key individuals in the community and presentations were made to various groups. Program benefits for the direct participants and the larger community were delineated. Particular emphasis was placed on the important role that evaluation plays in insuring that programs accomplish their aims and that scarce dollars are well spent. Individuals with demonstrated credibility in the community were enlisted to share their impressions based on in-depth discussions and review of our curriculum and/or feedback from their constituents who had participated in Project SANKOFA. To strengthen community ties, the SANKOFA program was implemented as a free community service for several organizations who were research sites.

5. Identify Research Sites/Develop Collaborative Relationships

The study sites were selected to permit both an exploratory test of the intervention's effectiveness within different youth populations, and as a replication across settings and populations. All study sites are located in the same neighborhood of an urban area in the northeast United States.

The principal investigator sent letters and subsequently scheduled meetings with administrators at organizations identified as potential study sites. The main issues discussed included: (1) the project aims, (2) the perceived need for a youth violence prevention program at the site, (3) the potential benefits of the project for the organization as well as to participants and the larger community, (4) past, ongoing, and planned efforts at the site and larger community that related to the aims of Project SANKOFA, and (5) the potential for the organization to meet the criteria for participation in the project. The principal investigator pledged to provide training at the end of the project to selected staff at the study sites so that each would have a means of continuing the SANKOFA program. Administrators were asked to either serve as, or designate a liaison to the project. A meeting schedule was established to insure ongoing exchange of information and problem-solving, as needed. A written affiliation agreement was formulated and signed by the principal investigator and chief operating officer at each study site, detailing the responsibilities of each. SANKOFA staff were allowed to spend time at each site during the project planning phase to become familiar with the daily schedule, building layout, key players, and to concretize logistical arrangements. Staff made an ongoing effort to establish and nurture relationships with office support and security staff. In addition, SANKOFA staff attended staff/faculty meetings at the research sites on a regular basis to make announcements, provide updates, and hear and respond to information/concerns relevant to project implementation.

Administrative staff at the study sites were generally busy, overloaded, and distracted by threatened lay-offs. Communications between administrators/designated liaisons and their staff/colleagues were sometimes delayed, resulting in slower than anticipated follow-up on essential decisions and/or tasks. In some instances, liaison persons made decisions different from those initially communicated by site administrators. The affiliation agreement proved to be useful for redirecting attention to the parameters initially agreed upon.

6. Select Intervention Schedule

To minimize unnecessary disruptions in implementation of the adolescent intervention, school and program calendars were secured so that realistic schedules could be planned. Staff inquired about the potential for scheduling additional events (e.g., testing, staff development, and teacher-parent conferences) that were not already listed on the calendars. Policies for weather cancellations were clarified. Information was secured regarding the number of students who are bussed as well as daily and seasonal attendance rates. Staff consulted with students about events that might interfere with group member attendance and secured very useful information. Taking this collective information into account, staff mapped out the dates for each intervention cycle; make-up dates were routinely included in each training schedule in the event sessions were canceled.

The initial 24-hour intervention is delivered in 12, two-hour sessions over a six week period. The group sessions are scheduled during the school day so that students do not miss the same academic subject twice in a week. The session length (2 hours) was selected on the premise that each session must be sufficiently long to help youth transition from pre-group activities, give adequate coverage to the topics introduced, actively engage youth, motivate behavioral change, and give them an opportunity to try out new behaviors between sessions. Another operating assumption is that fewer subjects will be lost if the program is brief but intensive.

In spite of varied efforts to minimize scheduling disruptions, it proved impossible to avoid disruptions due to reorganization of the school district. A large number of personnel changes were made in the district's central administration. Administrators at the three school sites were occasionally without choice with regard to modifying student schedules to respond to unexpected mandates (e.g., specific number of hours of preparation for minimum skills test).

7. Conduct Facilitator Training

The authors of the SANKOFA curriculum (both experienced trainers) involved the prospective SANKOFA group facilitators (trainees) in a multi-step training process. Formal classroom training covered the research aims and implementation plan, the findings from the initial focus groups, tips regarding behavioral management in groups, and the necessity of fidelity in curriculum implementation. The trainees reviewed the text of the curriculum and associated videos. Subsequently, the trainees and trainers reviewed and discussed videotapes of a pilot group facilitated by one of the trainers; the trainers offered consultation regarding content and process issues. Trainees were engaged in a self-assessment and discussion of issues likely to arise in their work with urban teens. The next phase involved apprentice training. In brief, each trainee co-facilitated a group with one of the two trainers. Debriefing was held after each session during which the trainees received consultation regarding their facilitation and the trainer responded to questions. Finally, the trainees conducted the SANKOFA intervention alone while the trainers observed. They received feedback at the end of each group session based on the trainer's direct observations.

8. Recruit Participants

Targeted youth are between the ages of 14 and 19 and must live within the designated ward of the city. Participation is voluntary. There are no other exclusionary criteria. Participants are recruited from the youth populations served by the study sites through a variety of strategies. Announcements are made by loudspeaker and fliers are distributed in classrooms, school assemblies, and the cafeteria. SANKOFA staff conduct brief orientation sessions consisting of a skit and a verbal overview during gym classes or other time periods specified by the administrators. Youth who indicate an interest are registered and advised that their participation is contingent on returning letters of informed consent with their own and their parent/guardian's signature. Consent forms are mailed to parents and phone calls were made by staff to encourage their return. As an incentive for timely return of consent forms, staff schedule a pizza party at the end of each recruitment week for those teens who had returned their signed consent forms by that day.

In their enthusiasm to attain a needed service for the teens in their targeted area, community-based organizations tended to overestimate the number of teens involved in their programs. Two organizations that were initially selected as research sites were eliminated once it became clear that their commitment to SANKOFA was based on a plan to increase teen enrollment in their ongoing programs. New project sites were quickly solicited.

A sizable number of youth consistently registered for the project, but failed to appear for the first SANKOFA session. In some instances, students, parents, and/or teachers were reluctant for teens to miss academic classes. In other instances, the initial interest appeared to be more a matter of following the crowd or inattention to the importance of returning the consent forms. A decision was made to both distribute informed consent letters directly to students and to mail them to the students' homes. After the first cohort of youth had completed the training, selected participants served as recruiters for the project.

9. Conduct PilotTest/Refine Implementation Plan

The recruitment methodology, assessment, and skills-training intervention were pilot-tested with a small group of youth from each of the participating research sites. Project staff conducted verbal discussions with the pilot group participants after each session to secure their input regarding possible changes in the intervention.

The pilot test confirmed our belief that group sizes should be limited to 10 to 12 participants. Participant and facilitator feedback led to clearer communication of key ideas, the shortening of some curriculum activities, simplification of the role play scripts and instructions, an increased awareness of the logistical issues that required attention at each study site (e.g., site staff intrusion), and revision of the evaluation survey. The process also clarified staff training guidelines (e.g., checking for code #s on each page of evaluation surveys) that needed to be reinforced or introduced. Lessons from the pilot test resulted in a substantial modification of our original plan in that the adolescent intervention during after-school hours was abandoned at all sites except the youth detention center.

10. Attendance and Subject Retention

Participant attendance and subject loss to the study were predictable concerns for several reasons. Adolescents typically are engaged in a variety of extra-curricular activities and interests that compete for their attention. Parents often depend upon them to contribute to household income, provide child care for younger siblings, and assist with the care of elderly family members. Some students required unanticipated, special academic assistance that required changes in their school schedules. Some students cope with ongoing instability in their lives by school avoidance. For others (e.g., students in alternative school), regular school attendance is not a priority. Also, it is not uncommon in lower socioeconomic communities for students to change residences and to transfer to new schools during the course of the school year.

Our original intention was to conduct the intervention immediately after the school day at those school sites where administrative approval was not granted for implementing SANKOFA during school hours. However, the attendance rate of "after school" participants during the pilot study and the first field test cycle (at the mainstream high school) had poorer attendance than expected. Students expressed concern about a lack of safety walking home without their usual peer group. Because the project funding did not permit staff to provide transportation and it was not possible to schedule the groups during the school day, this school was dropped from the research study. Our implementation plan was revised so that all training sessions at school sites were scheduled during regular school hours.

The group from the detention center posed unique concerns because of their unpredictable and varying lengths of stay at the center. Project SANKOFA staff assisted by the project liaison at the detention center, reviewed the folders of each detainee to determine the probability that interested youth would be at the facility for at least three months to complete the intervention. Nevertheless, subject loss was consistently high because of court appearances and transfers to other facilities. The targeted sample size was increased at each site and interventions were continued at the detention center despite the high rate of subject loss because there were no alternative means of accessing this sub-population for study.

SANKOFA staff made reminder phone calls to registered youth one to two days prior to the start of each intervention cycle. Refreshments were served at the beginning of each group session, across sites. A lottery drawing was also conducted at each site to recognize and encourage good attendance. To reduce subject loss due to change of address and phone numbers, SANKOFA staff requested that participants provide the addresses and phone numbers of several persons who would always know how to contact them for tracking purposes. Ultimately, there were still subjects who were lost to the data pool.

11. Insure Safety/Address Ongoing Exposure to Violence

Safety problems have further threatened adequate implementation of the SANKOFA research program. Across study sites, staff encountered repeated disclosures about weapon carrying among students and observed evidence of inadequate security. At one research site, lighting in the hallway outside of the group intervention rooms was grossly inadequate and emergency calling equipment was broken. Given the seriousness of these safety concerns, interventions were delayed and ultimately terminated at two sites for part of the second year of field testing to permit administrators time to address safety concerns.

There were occasions on which security staff coverage was inadequate at the youth detention facility. Staff encountered continuous changes in policies and procedures at this site as a result of the administration's effort to tighten security and address problems that arose on any given day (e.g., fight on a unit requiring restricted movement of detainees). At one point, for example, SANKOFA staff were advised that they would not be allowed to bring training equipment or supplies. Although this issue was resolved, it was typical of challenges that required staff time to insure continuation of the project on schedule. Consideration of site specific issues also meant that flexibility was required in various implementation procedures. For example, youth at the detention center were not allowed to be paid directly for survey completion; payments were deposited in the youth's accounts with the facility. While SANKOFA staff brought refreshments to each SANKOFA meeting at other research sites, security measures at the youth house dictated that the facility provide the refreshments.

Some personnel at the study sites were observed to have inadequate training to deal with various crises that arose. As circumstances dictated, SANKOFA staff responded to requests and assisted with various crises (e.g., suicidal threats). Project SANKOFA staff delayed the group intervention on several occasions in order to counsel group members following the tragic deaths of teens in their school or community. It was necessary and important to repeatedly reiterate to participating agencies; however, the SANKOFA staff's inability to assume such roles on an ongoing basis. The principal investigator underscored the need for administrators at the research sites to improve students' access to services by designating someone from their staff to develop an ongoing, active relationship with key community service organizations. SANKOFA staff also informed research site administrators about free training and consultation opportunities.

12. Develop Final Research Plan

The original research plan involved an experimental, repeated measures, delayed entry control group design. The plan was to randomly assign participants to either the intervention or the control group at the beginning of each cycle. However, adolescents were slow to return signed parental consent forms forcing delays in program implementation until an adequate number of youth returned parental permission forms. After several weeks delay, a decision was made to forego the experimental design in order to secure a sufficiently large sample of intervention participants. This change in plans resulted in a quasi-experimental research design comparing the intervention group to a purposefully recruited comparison group of adolescents from the same project sites. The comparison group is tested using the research questionnaires at intervals comparable to the intervention group's intake and posttest.

PRELIMINARY RESEARCH FINDINGS

The preliminary report of research findings from the ongoing project is based on an initial sample of 309 youth who participated in the SANKOFA adolescent training group interventions. These 309 youth were recruited from the youth detention center (35%), a community based organization serving high school drop-outs (21%), an alternative high school for behaviorally disordered youth (30%), a high school for classified youth (8%), and a mainstream high school (6%). The sample ranged in age from 15 to 21, was 70% male and 30% female, and predominantly African American (83%), Latino/Hispanic (8%), or Caribbean (2%).

Typical of inner city youth, subjects participating in SANKOFA reported high exposure to violence and were often involved in fights. Sixty-three percent of the participants reported they had been an active participant in a fight during the preceding three months, and 52% reported having injured someone during this same time period. Seventy-six percent (76%) felt they could protect themselves if physically attacked. This self-assurance was primarily attributable to the possession of weapons: 50% said they had carried a weapon in the past three months, usually a knife or a club. However, 30% said they had carried a hand gun in the previous three months, and one-half the sample reported carrying a gun at least once in their lives. In spite of their reliance on weapons for self-defense, the SANKOFA participants were not sure they could control their use. More than half (53%) said they weren't sure they could control their temper, and 55% weren't sure they could stay out of a fight; 75% reported their parents did not want them to fight or carry a weapon. Interestingly, these high levels of youth violence did not appear to correspond to high rates of drug use or to gang membership. Only 23% of the sample reported having taken part in a fight between gangs. Equally interesting, a majority reported living in their neighborhoods more than five years, with a third having lived there all their lives. Seventy-five percent said that there were at least one or two adults in their neighborhood they could count on for help, and 62% said they 'fairly often' or 'almost always' tried to do what their parent or guardian wanted. These low rates of gang membership and high rates of neighborhood support and family connectedness challenge the image of violent youth as alienated and at odds.

PARTICIPANT CHANGE

Four separate repeated-measure multiple analyses of variance (MANOVA) were conducted with blocks of outcome variables targeted by the intervention. The first MANOVA included three variables based on participant self-reports of violent behavior and violent tendencies: *Frequency of carrying weapons*, *self-control of aggressive impulses*, and *perpetrated harm*. The main effect for participant change over time was statistically significant for this block of variables ($F(1,111) = 9.16$; $p < .01$), with participants improving significantly on two of the included variables: *self-control of aggressive impulse* ($F(1,112) = 2.39$, $p < .02$) and *perpetrated harm* ($F(1,121) = 3.26$, $p < .001$).

A second repeated-measure MANOVA was conducted with the measures, *attitude toward weapons*, *susceptibility to social pressure* and *belief in ability to avoid violence*. This analysis did not reveal any overall significant change in participants over time, although there was a trend toward improvement in belief in ability to avoid violence.

A third MANOVA was conducted with three variables related to the emotional impact of exposure to violence (*anxiety*, *fear of victimization*, and *witness to violence*). The overall main effect for this analysis was statistically significant ($F(1,117) = 8.55$, $p < .01$), and attributable to one specific variable in the block: *witness to violence* ($F(1,119) = 3.93$, $p < .001$).

The fourth MANOVA included variables targeted by the project, but indirectly related to the occurrence of violence: *ethnic identity*, *drug or substance abuse*, and *parental affiliation*. There was no significant change on these variables over time for the sample as a whole.

VARIABLES PREDICTING PARTICIPANT REDUCTION IN PERPETRATED HARM

The practical significance of the MANOVA findings were explored through a discriminant function analysis ($X^2 = 26.67$; $p < .001$) comparing youth who did and did not inflict physical violence on others while participating in SANKOFA. Participant post-test responses to the item measuring *perpetrated harm* were dichotomized into *no harm* versus *any harm* groupings, and this new variable was entered as the dependent variable in the discriminant function analysis. Other variables for which there was significant improvement over time (or a trend toward significant improvement) were entered into the analysis as predictor variables to determine their relationship to the primary outcome variable *perpetrated harm*. These independent variables included *self-control of aggressive impulses*, *witness to violence*, and *belief in ability to avoid violence*. In addition, the new variable *anger* (designed during the second year of the project) and the third variable in the block of self-reports of aggressive behavior (*frequency of carrying weapons*) were included in the discriminant function analysis because of their theory-based potential for predicting *perpetrated harm*.

The results of the discriminant function analysis suggest that the obtained reduction in violent behavior within the SANKOFA participant sample is at least partly attributable to three mediating outcome variables targeted by the SANKOFA intervention: *Self-control, belief in ability to avoid violence*, and *frequency of carrying weapons.* Two predisposing variables also significantly predicted violent behavior: *self-reported* anger and the *frequency with which the individual had witnessed violence*. Participant post-test scores on these five variables correctly predicted the classification of 73% of the participants as those who either had (34%) or had not (66%) *shoved, slapped, hit, stabbed, or shot* someone during the intervention period.

EFFECTS ACROSS POPULATIONS

Separate repeated measure MANOVAs were performed for each of the four study sites to explore possible outcome differences across sites in the extent of participant change following SANKOFA, and to obtain an indication of the robustness of the main study findings (i.e., whether the findings were replicated at the site level of analysis, or whether the overall significant improvements could be attributed to pre-post differences at a single site). The preliminary findings are reassuring: The main study findings were replicated at the four sites which had sufficient samples to allow pre-post analyses.

CONCLUSION

The implementation of preventive intervention research in community settings is difficult at best. The SANKOFA research project has yielded both expected and unanticipated implementation challenges, requiring ongoing problem-solving to achieve the project's service and evaluation objectives and to insure the integrity of project findings. Like most prevention projects, SANKOFA's limited funding reduced the options available to avoid and address various implementation problems. The success of the field research has been heavily dependent upon the commitment, cooperation, and follow-through of community organizations. Unfortunately, those communities where the need for prevention programs is greatest are likely to have the least resources and present the greatest implementation problems. In spite of the challenges encountered, the preliminary findings of Project SANKOFA indicate that it is possible to design and implement a preventive intervention to effectively equip youths with the necessary life skills to reduce their risk for engaging in behaviors that compromise their safety and their lives.

REFERENCES

Ajzen, I. (1991). The theory of planned behavior. *Organizational Behavior and Human Decision Processes, 50*, 179-211.

Ajzen, I., & Fishbein, M. (1980). *Understanding attitudes and predicting social behavior*. Englewood Cliffs, NJ: Prentice-Hall.

Ajzen, I., & Madden, T. (1986). Prediction of goal-directed behavior: Attitudes, intentions, and perceived behavioral control. *Journal of Experimental Social Psychology, 22*, 453-474.

Bandura, A. (1989). Perceived self-efficacy. In V. M. Mays, G. W. Albee, & S. F. Schneider (Eds.), *Primary prevention of AIDS: Psychological approaches* (pp. 128-141). Newbury Park, CA: Sage.

Christoffel, K. K. (1990). Violent death and injury in US children and adolescents. *American Journal of the Diseases of Children, 144*, 697-706.

Fishbein, M., & Middlestadt, S. (1989). Using the theory of reasoned action as a framework for understanding and changing AIDS-related behaviors. In V. Mays, G. Albee, & S. Schenider (Eds.), *Primary prevention of AIDS: Psychological approaches* (pp. 93-110). Newbury Park, CA: Sage.

Kazdin, A. E. (1991). Prevention of conduct disorder. *The prevention of mental disorders: Progress, problems, and prospects*. Washington, DC: National Institute of Mental Health.

Madden, T. J., Ellen, P. S., & Azjen, I. (1992). A comparison of the theory of planned behavior and the theory of reasoned action. *Personality and Social Psychology Bulletin, 18*, 3-9.

National Center for Injury Prevention and Control. (1995). *10 Leading Causes of Death, 1992*. Atlanta, GA: Centers for Disease Control and Prevention.

O'Donnell L., Cohen S., & Hausman A. (1990). *The evaluation of community-based violence prevention programs*. Prepared for Forum on Youth Violence in Minority Communities: Setting the Agenda for Prevention, Atlanta, Dec.

Powell, K. E., & Hawkins, D. F., (Eds.) (1996). Youth Violence Prevention: Descriptions and Baseline Data from 13 Evaluation Projects. *American Journal of Preventive Medicine, 12*(5).

Successful Program Development Using Implementation Evaluation

Kathleen Bodisch Lynch
Susan R. Geller
Denise R. Hunt
Virginia Institute for Developmental Disabilities

Joseph Galano
Judith Semon Dubas
College of William and Mary

SUMMARY. Four methods used to enhance implementation of a resiliency-based early childhood substance abuse and violence prevention initiative are described. Project staff drew up formal agreements with participating programs to ensure administrative support for the

---

Address correspondence to: Kathleen Bodisch Lynch, Virginia Institute for Developmental Disabilities, P.O. Box 843020 VCU, Richmond, VA 23284-3020 (E-mail: klynch@saturn.vcu.edu). Correspondence concerning the Resilient Children Making Healthy Choices Project may be directed to Susan R. Geller, Project Director, at the same address (E-mail: sgeller@atlas.vcu.edu).

The authors gratefully acknowledge the work of the entire staff and consultant team of the RCMHC Project and the Virginia Institute for Developmental Disabilities, and their student assistants. They also thank the preschool administrators, teachers, and children for their cooperation and participation in this project.

This research was supported by grant 86872-103-94, funded from the Secretary of Public Safety, Office of the Governor of the Commonwealth of Virginia via the U. S. Drug-Free Schools and Communities Act.

[Haworth co-indexing entry note]: "Successful Program Development Using Implementation Evaluation." Lynch, Kathleen Bodisch et al. Co-published simultaneously in *Journal of Prevention & Intervention in the Community* (The Haworth Press, Inc.) Vol. 17, No. 2, 1998, pp. 51-64; and: *Program Implementation in Preventive Trials* (ed: Joseph A. Durlak, and Joseph R. Ferrari) The Haworth Press, Inc., 1998, pp. 51-64. Single or multiple copies of this article are available for a fee from The Haworth Document Delivery Service [1-800-342-9678, 9:00 a.m. - 5:00 p.m. (EST). E-mail address: getinfo@haworthpressinc.com].

intervention, provided high quality training for program implementers, used a participatory evaluation approach, and monitored implementation both directly and through practitioners' self-report. The contribution of each of these methods to fidelity of implementation is discussed, and implementation challenges are identified. The growth and success of the project demonstrates the utility of implementation evaluation data for ongoing program development and improvement. *[Article copies available for a fee from The Haworth Document Delivery Service: 1-800-342-9678. E-mail address: getinfo@haworth.com]*

Within the past decade there has been increased concern over the dramatic rise in the incidence of violence and substance abuse involving youth, particularly younger children (APA, 1993). While the extent, severity, and effects of involvement with violence and drugs vary, few children escape exposure altogether (Garbarino, Dubrow, Kostelny, & Pardo, 1992). Children who confront substance abuse and violence in their homes, schools, and communities are at increased risk of accepting these behaviors as normative. Even children of preschool age (three- and four-year-olds) have been observed to bring drug paraphernalia to school for show and tell, or to mimic rituals of substance use in their play (Hunt & Geller, 1996).

There is both a need and considerable support for designing and implementing preventive interventions for young children. Hawkins, Catalano, and Miller (1992) argued that "if the goal is to reduce drug abuse and its accompanying social and health problems among children at high risk, it is important to test preventive approaches that have successfully addressed risk factors present earlier in child development" (p. 97). Although preschool substance abuse prevention programs do exist, they are scarce in the literature, tend to have limited evaluation strategies, and frequently lack outcome data (Lecca & Watts, 1993).

As significant adults in children's lives, teachers have the opportunity to assist children in learning skills that will help them become resilient to life's adversities. While this potential role for early childhood professionals has been recognized (Slaby, Roedell, Arezzo, & Hendrix, 1995), typical training programs neither equip teachers to address the impact on children of societal problems such as violence and substance abuse, nor provide instruction on how to design and carry out prevention strategies in the classroom.

The Resilient Children Making Healthy Choices Project (RCMHC) addressed these dual needs for teacher training and classroom prevention practices by designing an intervention based on resiliency research. Cross-cultural studies have identified common characteristics of children who grow up to be resilient, that is, who overcome adverse life situations and develop into healthy, successful adolescents and adults. These characteristics have been described as: social competence, problem-solving abilities, autonomy, and a sense of purpose and belief in a bright future (e.g., Rutter, 1987; Werner, 1993). Environmental "protective factors" that elicit and foster resiliency in children include caring relationships, especially with trusted adults; high expectation messages; opportunities for meaningful participation and decision making; and drug-free, anti-violence norms (e. g., Benard, 1996; Garmezy, 1985). RCMHC's goal was to help adults enhance protective factors by creating safe and caring environments for young children, thereby nurturing children's development of resiliency.

KEY ELEMENTS OF PROGRAM IMPLEMENTATION

RCMHC used a school-based prevention model in which teachers and their assistants were trained to provide the intervention. This teacher-as-preventionist approach has been shown to have durable results in decreasing children's risk of future substance abuse (Botvin, Baker, Dusenbury, Botvin, & Diaz, 1995). RCMHC teachers presented prevention concepts and fostered resiliency skills by conducting a 42-lesson classroom prevention curriculum, and were encouraged to reinforce these concepts and skills in naturally occurring situations throughout each day.

Two elements essential to implementing the RCMHC intervention with integrity relate to *content* and *approach*. The content of the curriculum was derived by examining the literature describing characteristics of resilient individuals, identifying the specific skills that defined these characteristics, and then creating lessons to nurture these skills in young children. For example, the ability to think flexibly is one aspect of problem solving. To encourage the development of flexible thinking, project developers designed several lessons to introduce, teach, and practice brainstorming (i.e., generating as many different ideas as possible without critiquing them). Each curriculum lesson was aimed at strengthening children's skills related to one or more of the components of resiliency. Explicit written instructions explained how to introduce the lesson (setting the stage for learning), how to carry out the activities, how to use project materials, and how to process what occurred with the children by using indicated discussion questions. Teachers were directed to conduct the lessons as written, and to implement the curriculum in its entirety.

Effective delivery of the intervention also required teachers to use a facilitative approach to guide children in developing resiliency skills.

Teachers were to use this approach to enhance the protective factors in the environment over which the teacher had some control. That is, teachers carrying out the RCMHC intervention with integrity would interact with children in ways that demonstrated that they cared about the children, believed they were capable, expected them to succeed, and expected them to lead safe and healthy lifestyles. Specific skills characteristic of the facilitative approach included: helping children explore their ideas, validating children's feelings and experiences, showing respect and understanding, providing appropriate information about healthful and harmful choices, facilitating brainstorming of ideas, guiding problem solving, modeling healthy behavior, allowing children to choose self-control, and communicating clear, no-use norms.

Preliminary findings from a comprehensive process and outcome evaluation indicate that RCMHC was effective in improving preschool teachers' competencies in promoting children's resiliency-related behaviors (Dubas, Lynch, Galano, Geller, & Hunt, in press). This paper focuses on issues pertaining to evaluating and enhancing program implementation.

WHY BE CONCERNED ABOUT MONITORING IMPLEMENTATION?

Conducting exquisitely designed evaluations of social programs in the absence of information about how or whether conditions differ between "intervention" and "control" situations is an exercise of questionable value. Evaluators of preventive interventions often can neither totally control the administration and dosage of the independent variable (i.e., "the program"), nor eliminate extraneous influences that might differentially affect experimental and control groups during program trials. The notion that variation in implementation is important for the analysis and interpretation of outcome data is clear from studies that have found a relationship between quality of implementation and strength of outcomes achieved (see Durlak, this volume). Without implementation data, conclusions may be prematurely drawn about a program's apparent ineffectiveness when, in reality, inadequate implementation did not allow a valid test of the program (Scheirer & Rezmovic, 1982). The assumption that the intervention is being implemented as planned must be assessed systematically, rather than taken for granted. Moreover, since interventions both affect and are affected by the environments in which they are carried out, implementation is rarely a static, either/or situation (Garaway, 1995).

Rather, imperfect degrees of implementation usually occur (Durlak, this volume).

METHODS TO ENHANCE QUALITY OF PROGRAM IMPLEMENTATION

Four different methods were used by RCMHC to enhance quality of implementation. First, a memorandum of understanding that outlined the responsibilities and commitment of RCMHC and participating program sites was drawn up and signed by each party. Second, RCMHC provided intensive, high quality training to the teachers and instructional assistants who implemented the intervention. Third, the use of a participatory evaluation approach introduced project participants to basic concepts of program evaluation, giving them a sense of ownership and a better understanding of why it was important to carry out the intervention with fidelity. Fourth, quality of implementation was assessed both by direct observation and by teacher self-report.

Ensure Administrative Support

RCMHC entered into a memorandum of understanding (MOU) with each participating educational program. The MOU stipulated the expectations and responsibilities of each party to the agreement, and ensured that local program administrators provided the support needed at the intervention and comparison sites to carry out project implementation and/or evaluation activities. For instance, the MOU clearly specified that both the teacher and instructional assistant from each intervention classroom were required to participate in an initial 3-day training session and ongoing training and feedback sessions during the project year. Teachers were to implement all 42 lessons in the prevention curriculum, conducting approximately two lessons per week, and they were expected to share their impressions of the project's strengths and weaknesses both in writing and in group feedback sessions. Participating intervention and comparison sites were required to cooperate with the project evaluation, complete evaluation instruments in a timely fashion, and facilitate RCMHC staff's classroom observations. In return, RCMHC agreed to provide training and ongoing technical assistance, supply all needed project materials, pay for substitute teachers during participants' attendance at project training sessions, and reimburse teachers for RCMHC-related travel and meal expenditures.

Provide High Quality Training

As another means of enhancing fidelity of implementation, RCMHC provided teachers with intensive, high-quality training to convey both the "why" and the "how" of the teacher-as-preventionist model. In accordance with recommendations from adult learning theory, the training combined brief theoretical lectures, participatory and experiential activities, and modeled demonstrations of targeted skills and behaviors (Gioia & Sims, 1985). A review of key concepts from resiliency research and prevention theory provided teachers with a knowledge base and conceptual framework to organize their learning. Training in RCMHC's facilitative approach addressed such topics as active listening, responding to children's disclosure of sensitive issues, and techniques for guiding children's development of prosocial behavior, interpersonal problem solving, healthy decision making, and coping. To convey how to implement prevention strategies in the classroom, RCMHC staff demonstrated teaching techniques, conducted sample lessons from the curriculum, and provided structured opportunities for teachers to practice and strengthen their skills.

Use Participatory Evaluation

RCMHC's approach to evaluation used many features of participatory evaluation, in which program improvement and development are considered to be legitimate evaluation goals, and practitioners are valued partners (Cousins, 1996). In participatory evaluation, program stakeholders are involved in every phase of evaluation, from problem formulation, to instrumentation, to data collection and reporting. While the evaluator's expertise is employed in providing training, technical support, and quality control, conducting the study is seen as a shared responsibility.

Participatory evaluation strategies have been identified as particularly appropriate for resiliency programs (Benard, 1995). RCMHC sought teachers' input during the design and refinement of evaluation strategies, identification and pilot-testing of instruments, exploration of methods for collecting outcome data, and consideration of feasible ways to obtain longitudinal data. Teachers' feedback on RCMHC's training, curriculum, and materials was used to guide project modifications and improvements.

Monitor Implementation

Three different methods were employed to gather implementation data. Each method produced a different type, depth, and range of information to help staff understand how teachers actually implemented the RCMHC intervention in their classrooms.

Direct Observation. RCMHC staff visited each intervention classroom on two or three occasions to observe teachers implementing curriculum lessons and interacting with children. Staff used the project-developed 13-item Implementation Monitoring and Observation Form (IMOF) to rate teachers on skills targeted by the project training, such as supporting children's communication of ideas and feelings, facilitating children's problem solving and decision making, and modeling safe and healthy choices. Staff also assigned two global ratings to indicate the degree to which teachers: (a) used the approaches and techniques promoted by the project to foster resilience in children; and (b) effectively communicated the prevention message that the observed lessons were designed to convey.

Written Self Report. Teachers were asked to complete a Lesson Feedback Sheet (LFS) for each lesson. LFSs included brief rating scale items, Yes-No questions, and open-ended questions designed to gather information about teachers' perceptions of the lesson's effectiveness, children's reactions to and understanding of the lesson, and the ease of carrying out the lesson. Teachers also recorded how much of each lesson they completed, any problems they experienced, any changes they made, lesson length, and suggestions for improvements. Teachers mailed back packets of completed LFSs on a regular schedule. All written comments and quantitative data were compiled and reviewed by project staff.

Teacher Feedback Meetings. Another type of self-report data on implementation was obtained through evaluator-led group interviews with all teachers and instructional assistants. These videotaped sessions were conducted four times during the project year. Teachers were asked to share both their difficulties and successes when implementing the curriculum. Questions were posed to elicit teachers' perceptions of the project's strengths and weaknesses, and to identify any unclear methods and concepts. Because of the trusting relationship that had been established through the participatory evaluation approach, these feedback meetings yielded rich information about how the project developers' ideas and materials were translated–or not translated–into classroom implementation.

EFFECTIVENESS OF PROJECT METHODS FOR EVALUATING AND ENHANCING IMPLEMENTATION

Administrative Support

Drawing up a memorandum of understanding between RCMHC and each participating educational program was vital to obtaining the administrative support necessary to ensure fidelity of implementation. The MOU specified the educational administrator who served as contact person at each local site, thereby establishing lines of communication if RCMHC identified problems relating to teachers' compliance with participation in required training sessions or evaluation activities. The MOU also prohibited dissemination of project components without authorization from RCMHC. For example, one local program wanted to pass project materials on to a new teacher at the end of the school year, without having her complete the required RCMHC training. The MOU gave the RCMHC director the authority to require either that the new teacher be trained, or that the project materials be returned (they were returned). Thus, the MOU was an effective tool for enhancing fidelity of implementation.

Training

Teachers reported in the Teacher Feedback Meetings that RCMHC training was useful, relevant, applicable to their classrooms, and critically needed. In particular, they indicated that the conceptual framework derived from resiliency research helped them realize that they were already acting as preventionists, and provided guidance on how they could build on their existing strengths.

Teachers stated that the training influenced their teaching styles. For example, teachers frequently cited as particularly significant the training on how to decide "whose problem is it." They reported that if they resisted their natural impulse to intervene immediately when observing two children in conflict, stepped back, and let the children own the problem, the children frequently were able to generate and choose socially appropriate solutions. This approach to resolving conflict in the classroom was consistent with implementing the program with integrity, and is just one example of several areas of behavior change that teachers attributed to training. External observers' ratings validated the teachers' self-reports; intervention teachers scored significantly higher than comparison group teachers at posttest on observational measures of positive, supportive, and nurturing teacher-child interactions (Dubas et al., in press).

Participatory Evaluation

The participatory evaluation approach was helpful in establishing a genuine partnership between program developers (RCMHC staff) and program implementers (the teachers), imbuing a sense of shared responsibility for ongoing program development and improvement through collecting, reporting, and using evaluation data. This feeling of joint ownership was evident in the teachers' cooperation with evaluation procedures. Perhaps most remarkable was the 100% return rate of LFSs during the 1994-95 project period, representing a total of 420 completed forms mailed back by 10 teachers on a predetermined schedule over a 5-month period.

Teachers also demonstrated a heightened sensitivity to factors that might have a negative impact on RCMHC's ability to collect valid and reliable data. For example, after having completed ratings of their children using an instrument designed to identify children's coping strategies, teachers reported that the items were difficult to answer at pretest; they believed they needed to know the children better before they could rate their coping styles accurately. Teachers actually recommended using their own time to re-do the ratings after several weeks, and all teachers participating in the project cooperated in completing these additional assessments.

Finally, because of the variability in implementing curriculum lessons that was observed during monitoring visits (see Table 1), the RCMHC evaluator took the opportunity during one of the Teacher Feedback Meetings to review and elaborate on the rationale for requiring teachers to adhere to the lessons' design. This discussion was not originally planned and would not have occurred if the project had not been collecting implementation data. Teachers' follow-up questions revealed that they comprehended both the importance of implementation fidelity, and the effects that lack of fidelity would have on the quality of the evaluation. For example, teachers asked whether they could use skills that were to be introduced to the children in later lessons in the curriculum if the skills were appropriate at an earlier time. They also sought guidance on how to report data on children who entered their program after the RCMHC curriculum had begun, since these children did not get the full implementation. Thus, it was apparent that teachers better understood that variability in implementation could compromise the usefulness of evaluation data for program improvement purposes.

Implementation Monitoring

The use of direct observation of implementation of a sample of lessons from the curriculum allowed RCMHC staff to ascertain the extent to which teachers implemented the intervention as intended and to identify trouble spots such as misunderstanding of key concepts, difficulties with applying and generalizing RCMHC approaches and techniques, and problems with using project curriculum and materials. These monitoring visits yielded both quantitative and qualitative data on fidelity of implementa-

TABLE 1. Means for Individual Teachers on Three Measures of Implementation

	Measure		
Teacher number	Implementation Monitoring and Observation Form (IMOF)[a]	Integrity of approach[b]	Integrity of content[b]
1	50.00	6.00	5.67
2	59.67	8.67	5.67
3[c]	64.50	10.00	8.00
4	53.67	8.00	6.00
5	56.33	8.33	9.67
6[c]	47.50	7.00	5.00
7	53.33	9.00	10.00
8	54.00	7.00	7.33
9[c]	52.00	8.50	10.00
10[c]	57.50	9.00	10.00
M	54.85	8.15	7.73
SD	4.90	1.18	2.07

Note. Unless indicated otherwise, values are means of ratings made during 3 observations.

[a]13-item rating scale; maximum score = 65.

[b]Single-item rating; maximum score = 10.

[c]Teachers received 2 observations.

tion. Data from the 13-item IMOF revealed that teachers varied in the degree to which they demonstrated the facilitative skills promoted through RCMHC training (see Table 1). Mean total scores on the IMOF, averaged over the number of observations made per teacher, ranged from a low of 47.5 to a high of 64.5 (maximum score = 65). The single-item global ratings reflected greater variation in fidelity to content than fidelity to approach. Even the teacher who received nearly the maximum rating on the IMOF, and got the top rating on fidelity of approach, did not get the highest rating on fidelity of content. The RCMHC developers' concern about the importance of implementation integrity was supported by the finding of a modest positive correlation between fidelity of implementation as measured by the IMOF and child outcomes as captured by teacher ratings of child behavior (Dubas et al., in press).

Moreover, qualitative data obtained through the monitoring visits helped staff to identify specific implementation difficulties. For example, a problem related to fidelity of approach was observed when several teachers had difficulty conducting successful brainstorming lessons. They might allow one child to continue generating ideas without limit, while the other children in the group began to lose interest or become disruptive. Subsequently, staff allocated time in one of the scheduled training and feedback sessions to review the concept of brainstorming and demonstrate its appropriate use.

Problems with presentation of RCMHC content were also noted. In some cases, teachers competently led children through the different activities that comprised a lesson from the prevention curriculum, but either did not introduce the lesson as directed, or failed to use the process questions that were included as facilitation guides. As a result, children did not receive the prevention message. Staff addressed this issue by providing additional training, revising materials to highlight the key points of each lesson, and creating an overlay page for each lesson that summarized essential implementation information.

Data from implementation observations were complemented by teachers' self-reports on the LFSs and during Teacher Feedback Sessions. The LFSs, which contained detailed comments from each teacher on each lesson, provided a breadth of information, and the discussions at the Teacher Feedback Meetings provided depth. Finally, at the end of the project year, teachers were invited to share their formatting and design ideas with RCMHC staff to make the curriculum more teacher-friendly and easy to use. Teachers who continued with the project the next year saw many of their suggestions incorporated into the revised materials.

CHALLENGES TO MAINTAINING FIDELITY

Despite having in place several features designed to enhance implementation fidelity, RCMHC found that when testing a preventive intervention in community-based preschool settings, there were factors over which the project had little or no control. One of the most difficult problems to address was personnel changes, such as loss of instructional assistants from the intervention classrooms and replacement of them with aides who had not received the project's training, reassignment of intervention teachers to different classrooms during the course of the project, and teachers' illness-related extended absences from the classroom. Administrators did not always remember to communicate these personnel changes in time for RCMHC staff to take action to provide training or support to enhance continued fidelity of implementation.

An additional challenge to implementation was the natural variation in teaching skills among participants. For instance, teachers who lacked basic classroom management skills did not suddenly acquire them during the course of the project. Difficulties with maintaining children's attention interfered with these teachers' abilities to convey the messages of the preventive intervention effectively. RCMHC staff are considering whether additional training modules devoted to strengthening classroom management skills need to be developed and offered.

Finally, the rapidly growing demand for the intervention challenged the project's ability to be responsive to unmet needs without losing control over the quality of implementation. RCMHC's decision to disseminate its curriculum and materials only in conjunction with teachers' full participation in project training posed two sets of problems. First, some preschools found it financially and programmatically difficult to release both the classroom teacher and instructional assistant to attend the required introductory training. Second, RCMHC's staff resources limited the number of teachers who could be trained. To address these issues, staff have been investigating the feasibility of creating a series of training videotapes, using teleconferencing for training and technical assistance, increasing the pool of qualified RCMHC trainers, and training local program personnel to monitor implementation and provide technical assistance.

CONCLUSION

RCMHC employed four methods to enhance fidelity of implementation of its preschool prevention initiative: (a) exchanging a memorandum of understanding between RCMHC and local program sites; (b) providing high quality training; (c) using a participatory evaluation approach; and (d) monitoring implementation through classroom observation and teacher self-report. Project staff responded to identified implementation problems in a timely fashion, revamped training sessions, and made changes in project materials to enhance fidelity of implementation. Implementation issues outside the project's control were documented to allow their impact on outcomes to be analyzed.

Carefully observing, assessing, and monitoring implementation in the context of a comprehensive, ongoing evaluation of the intervention was critical to the successful development of RCMHC. Implementation data were used to revise and reshape the intervention in a continuing cycle of "develop-implement-evaluate-improve." Future RCMHC research will examine the effects of systematically varying key dimensions of implementation to determine more accurately the relationship between implementation variables and teacher and child outcomes. Such documentation will help adopting programs weigh the benefits they can expect against the requirements of adhering to fidelity of implementation. As RCMHC continues to grow and is disseminated more widely, project staff are beginning to explore creative ways to ensure fidelity of implementation through the increased use of technology and local staff training.

REFERENCES

American Psychological Association. (1993). Violence & youth: Psychology response. *Volume I: Summary Report of the American Psychological Association Commission on Violence and Youth*. New York, NY: Sol Goldman Charitable Trust.

Benard, B. (1995). Fostering resilience in children. *ERIC Digest*. Urbana, IL: ERIC Clearinghouse on Elementary and Early Childhood Education.

Benard, B. (1996, Winter). From research to practice: The foundations of the resiliency paradigm. *Resiliency in Action*, 7-11.

Botvin, G. J., Baker, E., Dusenbury, L., Botvin, E. M., & Diaz, T. (1995). Long-term follow-up results of a randomized drug abuse prevention trial with a white middle-class population. *Journal of the American Medical Association*, *273*, 1106-1112.

Cousins, J. B. (1996). Consequences of researcher involvement in participatory evaluation. *Studies in Educational Evaluation*, *22*, 3-27.

Dubas, J. S., Lynch, K. B., Galano, J., Geller, S., & Hunt, D. (in press). Preliminary evaluation of a resiliency-based preschool substance abuse and violence prevention project. *Journal of Drug Education*.

Durlak, J. A. 1998. Why program implementation is important. *Journal of Prevention & Intervention in the Community, 17(2)*.

Garaway, G. B. (1995). Participatory evaluation. *Studies in Educational Evaluation*, *21*, 85-102.

Garbarino, J., Dubrow, N., Kostelny, K., & Pardo, C. (1992). *Children in danger: Coping with the effects of community violence*. San Francisco: Jossey-Bass.

Garmezy, N. (1985). Stress-resistant children: The search for protective factors. In J. E. Stevenson (Ed.), *Recent research in developmental psychopathology* (pp. 213-233). Oxford: Pergamon Press.

Gioia, D. A. & Sims, H. P. (1985). Videotapes and vicarious learning: A technology for effective training. In L. D. Goodstein & J. W. Pfeiffer (Eds.), *The 1985 Annual: Developing Human Resources* (pp. 155-168). San Diego, CA: University Associates.

Hawkins, J. D., Catalano, R. F., & Miller, J. Y. (1992). Risk and protective factors for alcohol and other drug problems in adolescence and early childhood:

Implications for substance abuse prevention. *Psychological Bulletin, 112*, 64-105.

Hunt, D., & Geller, S. (1996). When drug abuse issues enter the classroom. *National Head Start Association Journal, XV*(2), 21-23.

Lecca, P. J. & Watts, T. D. (1993). *Preschoolers and substance abuse: Strategies for prevention and intervention*. Binghamton, NY: The Haworth Press, Inc.

Rutter, M. (1987). Psychosocial resilience and protective mechanisms. *American Journal of Orthopsychiatry, 57*, 316-331.

Scheirer, M. A., & Rezmovic, E. L. (1982). *Measuring the degree of program implementation: A methodological review*. Rockville, MD: Westat.

Slaby, R. G., Roedell, W. C., Arezzo, D., & Hendrix, K. (1995). *Early violence prevention: Tools for teachers of young children*. Newton, MA: Education Development Center.

Werner, E. E. (1993). Risk, resilience, and recovery: Perspectives from the Kauai longitudinal study. *Development and Psychopathology, 5*, 503-515.

Design and Implementation of Parent Programs for a Community-Wide Adolescent Alcohol Use Prevention Program

Carolyn L. Williams
Cheryl L. Perry
University of Minnesota

SUMMARY. Project Northland is a comprehensive community trial designed to evaluate programs for the primary prevention of alcohol-related problems during adolescence. It uses a community-wide model, that includes both demand and supply reduction techniques. The first phase of Project Northland (grades 6-8) was completed with the effective implementation of multiple, complementary programs including a multi-year social behavioral curriculum, intensive parental involvement components, peer leadership opportunities, and community-level changes through the formation of local task forces. This article describes the process used for developing and implementing the comprehensive parent interventions used during the first phase of the research, highlighting the elements that led to the successful implementation of the programs with very high participa-

Address correspondence to: Carolyn L. Williams, Division of Epidemiology, School of Public Health, University of Minnesota, 1300 South Second Street, Suite 300, Minneapolis, MN 55454-1015.

[Haworth co-indexing entry note]: "Design and Implementation of Parent Programs for a Community-Wide Adolescent Alcohol Use Prevention Program." Williams, Carolyn L., and Cheryl L. Perry. Co-published simultaneously in *Journal of Prevention & Intervention in the Community* (The Haworth Press, Inc.) Vol. 17, No. 2, 1998, pp. 65-80; and: *Program Implementation in Preventive Trials* (ed: Joseph A. Durlak, and Joseph R. Ferrari) The Haworth Press, Inc., 1998, pp. 65-80. Single or multiple copies of this article are available for a fee from The Haworth Document Delivery Service [1-800-342-9678, 9:00 a.m. - 5:00 p.m. (EST). E-mail address: getinfo@haworthpressinc.com].

tion rates by parents, their young adolescents, teachers, and community members. *[Article copies available for a fee from The Haworth Document Delivery Service: 1-800-342-9678. E-mail address: getinfo@haworth.com]*

Alcohol is the drug of choice for American adolescents, despite it being illegal for virtually all high school students and half the college-aged population (Johnston, O'Malley, & Bachman, 1993). It is a licit drug which allows for the modeling of health compromising behaviors by parents and other important adults in adolescents' lives. Parents, upon learning that their children are drinking, rather than using other drugs, often express relief, and this relative lack of concern suggests that adolescents' current alcohol-centered behaviors fit prevailing social norms and expectations about their alcohol use (Thomas, 1992). Widespread use of alcohol during adolescence is a significant public health problem in this country, accounting for a substantial portion of the total morbidity and mortality during adolescence (e.g., NIAAA, 1994; "Trends in Drug and Alcohol Use," 1993; Wagenaar & Perry, 1994).

Obviously, underage drinking can not be viewed as a single behavior with a simple cause, easily amenable to change. Rather, research suggests that programs with the greatest likelihood of reducing underage drinking and its related problems are those with multi-level interventions that target both individual behavior and environmental change (e.g., Dryfoos, 1993; Wagenaar & Perry, 1994). Project Northland, the largest community trial in the United States focusing on the primary prevention of alcohol-related problems during adolescence, is an example of the newer intervention strategies using a community-wide model that utilizes both demand and supply reduction techniques (Perry et al., 1993). The Project Northland interventions include school-based programs using a multi-year social behavioral curriculum, an intensive parental involvement component, peer leadership opportunities, as well as community task forces focusing on reducing adolescent access to alcohol. Project Northland is an ongoing study with two distinct phases, one focusing on early adolescence (1991-1994), now completed (Perry et al., 1993; 1996), and another that is in progress and covers the cohort's high school years (1995-1999). The National Institute on Alcohol Abuse and Alcoholism (NIAAA) has funded Project Northland researchers to continue developing interventions and evaluating their impact until the cohort graduates in 1998.

The Project Northland research design uses school districts randomized to intervention or reference conditions and implements a multi-level intervention program designed to change factors predictive of the onset of alcohol use (e.g., parent-child communication about parents' disapproval of underage drinking, peer influences to drink and students' ability to resist those influences, alcohol use norms, and students' access to alcohol in their communities). At the end of the first three years of the study, the Project Northland interventions were effective during early adolescence in reducing alcohol use, reducing the combination of cigarette and alcohol use, increasing parent-child communication about the consequences of drinking, changing many reasons perceived by adolescents for their alcohol use, reducing peer norms and peer influences to use, and introducing skills to resist peer influences (Perry et al., 1996). The larger social environment, particularly adolescents' access to alcohol in the community, was not impacted during the first phase of Project Northland.

The purpose of this article is to describe the Project Northland interventions for early adolescence, highlighting the development and implementation of the parent components. All Project Northland interventions are integrated and designed to facilitate change in the social environment of young people by giving a strong "no use" message. The Project Northland parent programs are part of this integrative intervention strategy and are seen as necessary, but not sufficient, behavior change strategies.

Underage drinking occurs primarily outside of school hours when parents are responsible for the young person's well-being. Various parent behaviors have been studied as predictors of adolescents' alcohol use, including moderate parental drinking (e.g., Brook, Whiteman, Gordon, Nomura, & Brook, 1986; Peterson, Hawkins, Abbott, & Catalano, 1994). Although others have not found an association with parental modeling of alcohol use (e.g., Ary, Tildesley, Hops, & Andrews, 1993), Peterson and colleagues (1994) suggest that the effect of parents' drinking may be mediated by family management practices and proscriptions against involving children in adult drinking (e.g., having children open or serve alcoholic beverages). Toomey, Williams, Perry, Murray, Dudovitz, and Veblen-Mortenson (1997) conclude, after a review of the literature, that the likelihood of the onset of underage drinking may be reduced if (1) parents have consistent rules against underage drinking and communicate their disapproval of teen alcohol use to their children; (2) parents actively monitor their children's activities and spend time with them; and (3) children are not allowed to consume alcohol with their parents. The Project Northland parent components were developed to target these predictive factors associated with the onset of underage drinking. Given the relationship of the parent component to the rest of the Project Northland interventions, it is important that they be presented within the context of the other intervention components.

PROJECT NORTHLAND PARTICIPANTS AND INTERVENTION PROGRAMS

Project Northland is being conducted in northeastern Minnesota in mostly rural, lower middle-class to middle-class communities. The recruitment of communities for Project Northland has been documented elsewhere (Perry et al., 1993). The primary study cohort is the Class of 1998 in 24 school districts that were systematically recruited and randomly assigned to the intervention condition (n = 10) or reference condition (n = 10). The students were sixth graders at baseline in the fall of 1991 (n = 2,351). Of these students, 94% were white and 5.5% were American Indians (Perry et al., 1996).

All Project Northland interventions were based on social learning theory and each year had a different social behavioral curricula. In sixth grade, the program was called Slick Tracy; the seventh grade program was Amazing Alternatives!; and the eighth grade program was PowerLines. This allowed us to redefine the intervention as the students passed through the grade levels and paralleled our hypotheses about developmentally appropriate interventions. We started intervening with young adolescents within their families, progressed to their peer groups, and ended the early adolescent phase in eighth grade with interventions targeted to their larger social environment.

Each year the intervention had three major components: school-based programs, parent involvement/education programs, and community task force activities. The primary focus of the sixth grade intervention was a home-based program that was administered as homework assignments from the school. It was designed to structure links between young adolescents and their parents by facilitating communication about alcohol use, and guiding parents to establish no-use rules, and appropriate consequences for breaking the rules. The seventh grade program primarily focused on skills development for dealing with peers and encouraged positive peer group influences. The eighth grade intervention empowered young people to create healthy changes in their environments by teaching them to look beyond the individual and school for influences in the community related to underage drinking. The community-based interventions began during seventh grade with the formation and training of task forces as primary mechanisms for community-wide action and continued throughout the intervention period.

PARENT PROGRAM DEVELOPMENT

Previous research involving parents in health promotion programs guided our efforts in program development. For example, other efforts to recruit and maintain parents in health education programs have been hampered by recruitment difficulties, poor attendance, high drop-out rates, or not attracting those parents whose children are at higher risk for alcohol or other drug use (e.g., Harding, Apsler, & Walsh, 1989; Klitzner, Gruenewald, & Bamberger, 1990; Perry, Crockett, & Pirie, 1987). A telephone survey asking parents' opinions about preferred parent education methods for nutrition topics found strong preferences for short interventions in the home, rather than programs at school or other locations (Perry et al., 1989): ranked from most to least preferred were behavioral tip sheets (75% reported interest); worksheets and homework from school that required parent involvement (67%); informational brochures (42%); phone calls about the topic (39%); and parent education nights (15%). Perry and colleagues (1989) demonstrated the feasibility of home-based programs for nutrition education and others have shown promising results for alcohol and other drugs (e.g., Pentz et al., 1989; Werch, Young, Clark, Garrett, Hooks, & Kersten, 1991).

All our parent involvement and educational materials were designed to enhance participation rates by being engaging, creative, and fun. Multiple strategies for involving parents were developed over the three years. Although the Slick Tracy Home Team was implemented as a required homework assignment, completion of its activities was reinforced with fun activities and incentives. A more traditional newsletter approach was also begun in sixth grade. Parents were recruited as volunteers to be peer group facilitators for the alternative activities that were developed by peer leaders in the various schools, beginning during the seventh grade program (Komro, Perry, Veblen-Mortenson, & Williams, 1994). Parents were also a major source of recruitment for community task forces, whose goal was to influence change at the community level by working on a supply reduction strategy. In seventh grade, we had a direct mailing of a series of four educational booklets to the parents of each student in the intervention communities (Toomey et al., 1997). For eighth grade we invited parents to attend "It's My Party," a play produced in each community.

A similar development process was used for all Project Northland parent interventions during early adolescence (e.g., Slick Tracy Home Team, Amazing Alternatives Home Program, and "It's My Party") and took place during the six to 12 months before the program was scheduled for implementation. The principal investigators of the study (Perry and Williams) identified and supervised various teams to develop these interventions. Fortunately, we maintained a stable core group throughout the intervention period that included a writer and curriculum specialist experienced in health promotion school-based interventions; as well as an intervention coordinator who was responsible for program implementation. A graphic artist was hired as a consultant to the various teams to provide age-appropriate and appealing illustrations for the educational materials. Doctoral students and others completed the various writing teams each year. Brainstorming sessions, informed by reviews of the literature and expert consultants, were used to select behavior change goals and to develop ideas for writing the programs.[1]

Focus groups with parents provided feedback about each team's proposed topics, as well as suggestions directly from parents about their perceptions of other information to include, and possible barriers to program implementation (e.g., time constraints, student resistance). Parents verified our beliefs that home-based sessions should take no longer than half an hour per week. Separate focus groups were also held with young adolescents who were asked to review materials for their attractiveness, age-appropriateness, and relevance to their lives, as well as to provide content suggestions. About half of the young adolescents told us that they did NOT want to talk with their parents about alcohol use, but all parents agreed the topic was important for family discussions, and welcomed suggestions about how to have successful conversations with their children. The focus groups with adolescents corroborated our views that fun and appealing materials were necessary to overcome student and parent discomfort and enhance participation.

Program materials (e.g., activity booklets for families and teacher training manuals) were drafted initially by the curriculum specialist and/or other researchers, and then reviewed and edited individually by team members. Final editing and approval were done by the principal investigators, who evaluated the materials for cultural and gender sensitivity. Care was also taken to ensure that the materials could be used by single parent families without potentially offensive assumptions about who are (or are not) family members. This process resulted in first drafts of the materials that were submitted to at least two more pilot test evaluations before being implemented in the intervention communities of Project Northland.

The initial "real world" pilot evaluations of the two primary Project Northland parent interventions (i.e., Slick Tracy and Amazing Alternative! Home Program) were completed with a "five-family pilot study." The first pilot test of the eighth grade parent intervention, a theater production, was somewhat different and is described below. The five families were a convenience sample selected from acquaintances of team members who had children in the targeted grades and lived in the Minneapolis area. After the initial contact and agreement to participate, the five families were sent the program materials by a team member who was not acquainted with them. The families were asked to read the materials and participate in the activities. At the end of each week, the parents were interviewed on the telephone and filled out a short written evaluation of the activities. Questions included what was liked and disliked about the materials, whether or not the content was helpful, how long it took and if the length was a problem, success in promoting discussion, and comments about the materials' tone, style, format, and content. Intervention materials were then revised based on information from the five-family pilot studies.

The second pilot tests of intervention materials were completed using approximately 80 students from four classrooms in a parochial school located in Mankato, Minnesota, a small community approximately 90 miles from the Twin Cities. Project Northland researchers observed all classroom sessions, met with teachers, students, and parents to learn how the program worked when implemented through a classroom setting. The final versions of the intervention materials were then prepared, and based on actual observations and comments from students, teachers, and parents. In some cases, the changes made after this pilot test were so substantive that another pilot test was undertaken in the fall with a new class of the parochial school students.

Because the eighth grade parent involvement program was a live theater production, the five-family pilot test was substituted for a pilot theater production. The Project Northland team collaborated with the Child's Play Theater Company of Minneapolis to develop a script and train actor-educators to produce a play in each of our intervention schools in northern Minnesota. One pilot test of this production was completed in Minneapolis with eighth grade actors recruited from the theater company, and the script and training were revised. Then the production was tested at the Mankato school that had taken part in our other pilot tests.

Slick Tracy Home Program. Project Northland began with the Slick Tracy Home Team Program in sixth grade. By beginning the primary prevention program in the home, we immediately enlisted parents as partners. The sixth grade intervention gave parents a first hand look at the rationale for primary prevention, along with our goals and objectives: promoting the health of youth by delaying or preventing onset of alcohol use, as well as reducing the amount of alcohol use by young adolescents. We believed that parents would readily accept these goals for their 12-year old children, and recognized that there might not be as widespread acceptance of our program goals if we began a prevention program with high school students instead.

The Slick Tracy Home Team Program was a four session home-based program administered through booklets from classrooms to the families of the cohort (Williams et al., 1995). The activity booklets included a comic narrative featuring the adventures of a detective named Slick Tracy and his partner, Breathtest Mahoney. These two adolescent characters served as positive role models and relayed the themes of the weekly booklets through an adventure. The theme for Week 1 was to present factual information on why underage drinking is a significant public health problem and encouraged parents and teens to communicate about underage drinking. Week 2 focused on modeling, including alcohol advertising, as well as parents as role models. Week 3 covered peer pressure and parent strategies to know their child's friends in order to combat negative peer group influences. Week 4 focused on the consequences of drinking and developing effective family guidelines about underage drinking.

Each of the weekly booklets had a similar format which included the comic narrative with the introduction of the theme for the week; two activities for parents and sixth graders to complete together; an activity for the student, "Private I," to encourage further thinking about the weekly theme; and a newsletter for parents, Northland Notes for Parents (Williams et al., 1995). The activities were designed to take no longer than 15 or 20 minutes of the family's time and could be completed any time during the week they were sent home. Home scorecards were returned to school each week and records were maintained on a scoreboard prominently displayed in the classroom. Incentives in the form of neon-colored shoe laces and pens were used to reinforce completion of the booklets. We also encouraged classroom teachers who introduced their own incentives, like a pizza party, for 100% participation. Coordinators based in the local schools monitored the classroom scoreboards and volunteered to work with any student who was having difficulty completing the activities at home.

The activity booklets were introduced in the classroom by elected peer leaders (n = 318) who were trained in two hour sessions by the local community coordinators and Minneapolis staff. Classroom teachers (n = 54) had been trained in a four hour session the previous week. Peer leaders, facilitated by their classroom teachers, explained to their classmates what was to be done with parents and focused on how fun the activity would be to increase the likelihood of high participation rates. The Slick Tracy Home Team Program was implemented in 53 classrooms across 14 school districts with 1,322 sixth graders and their families. Overall, 90% of our families completed at least one booklet, with 75% of them completing most or all of the booklets, defined as three or four (Williams et al., 1995). Fifty percent of the American Indian families completed most or all of the booklets. We also had a high completion rate for those young people already experiencing school and/or family problems, as measured by the MMPI-A (Williams et al., 1995).

The sixth grade program also included a Slick Tracy Fun Night at the school and in order to increase parent attendance, all children were involved as presenters of poster projects completed in pairs in their classrooms (Williams et al., 1995). Slick Tracy Fun Nights were held in each of the intervention schools for students and their families. Community leaders and representatives from law enforcement were invited to attend. Fifty-seven percent of the students attended the Fun Night, with almost all of them coming with at least one parent (51%). American Indian families were no less likely to attend the events than were white families (Williams et al., 1995).

In addition to the quantitative evaluation of participation in Slick Tracy's weekly activities and the family evening event (Williams et al., 1995), we also conducted focus groups with students identified by the classroom scoreboard and school coordinators as completing zero or one booklet with their parents. Interestingly, these young people were clearly exposed to the program's content as they could identify the various characters and themes the program was designed to convey. Although they did not benefit from having parents reinforcing the program's messages by developing family guidelines against underage drinking, they were not excluded entirely from the program, given the classroom and peer leader components, efforts of the community coordinators, and the inherent appeal of the comic narratives for this age level.

Amazing Alternatives! Program. The Amazing Alternatives! program for seventh grade was primarily an eight session peer classroom program. In their classrooms, students learned from their peers why kids their age begin to drink; influences from peers, older teens, and advertising; and skills to resist those influences. The peer leadership component of our intervention was increased significantly during seventh grade and the work of the community task forces continued. The seventh grade parent involvement components supplemented the Amazing Alternatives! school-based activities with (1) an evening event at the schools in the fall; (2) four activity booklets directly mailed to parents (Toomey et al., 1997); (3) continued opportunities for parents to participate as adult volunteers for peer-led extra-curricula activities (Komro et al., 1994); (4) continued distribution of the newsletter, *Northland Notes for Parents*; and (5) continued opportunities to serve as community task force volunteers, who were encouraged to work on supply reduction strategies.

The seventh grade school-based programs were kicked off with the Amazing Alternatives! Awesome Autumn Party held in each school. At this party, we modeled ways in which seventh graders could have fun without using alcohol by developing 13 games and other activities. At each Awesome Autumn Party, a separate section was set aside for parents to meet and talk. In this section, our Project Northland coordinators mingled informally with the parents and we provided discussion questions related to underage drinking for them to consider. As with the sixth grade evening event, community members were involved in these parties. Members of the local law enforcement served alcohol-free punch and gave out the recipes. Approximately 1,700 people at 20 different schools attended these parties in the intervention communities.

The Amazing Alternatives! Home Program (Toomey et al., 1997) continued the parent education program begun in sixth grade, with four booklets mailed directly to the parents. It was a supplementary intervention for seventh grade. Unlike the Slick Tracy Home Program, it was completely voluntary and not incorporated as homework assignments because the primary focus of the curriculum was peer influences and it was not feasible to use classroom time to implement a home program as well. Each of the four booklets had 2 parts including a section to be read by parents, followed by a discussion activity to be completed by parents and their seventh grader. The booklets provided guidelines for discussions about (1) alcohol-related situations faced by seventh graders; (2) development of family rules and consequences about underage drinking; (3) alcohol-related messages on television; and (4) ways parents can encourage seventh graders to socialize in their homes (Toomey et al., 1997). Because the program was voluntary, participants were eligible for a grand prize drawing by returning post cards indicating booklet completion for a trip to the Twin Cities (on average about 200 miles from the program communities).

The Home Program was evaluated to determine whether (1) a sufficient number of parents participated, (2) if participation in the program promoted family discussions or altered parenting behaviors, and (3) whether students whose parents participated reported less alcohol consumption (Toomey et al., 1997). We had two measures of participation, one involved parents voluntarily returning postcards upon completion of each booklet and the second was a telephone survey of 50% of the parents of the cohort. Although both measures were designed to estimate parent participation, they produced different rates, with 33% of the parents returning postcards indicating completion of at least one booklet, and 50% of the telephone survey parents indicating completion of at least one booklet. However, both estimates indicate that fewer parents participated in the seventh grade direct mailing activities, compared with the homework assignments in sixth grade (Williams et al., 1995). Even so, participation in the Amazing

Alternatives! Home Program was much higher than typical classroom-based parent education programs scheduled away from the home (Crockett et al., 1989; Harding et al., 1989), suggesting that a direct mailing intervention may reach more parents. Direct mailings to parents may be viable as adjunct interventions, particularly when school time is not available (or if the health education information is too sensitive) to facilitate the homework assignment approach that has the highest rates of participation (Toomey et al., 1997).

The evaluation of the Home Program booklets revealed that they were useful tools for promoting family discussions about underage drinking and increasing students' perceptions about their family's rules and consequences concerning alcohol use (Toomey et al., 1997). Other targeted parenting behaviors (e.g., increased monitoring of child's activities) did not show an intervention effect, nor did students whose parents' reported participation show lower drinking rates. However, since all subjects, both participants and nonparticipants in the Home Program booklets, were exposed to most other Project Northland interventions, the effects of the Home Program had to be large enough to be detected above the effects of the rest of Project Northland (Toomey et al., 1997). Project Northland's research design did not allow a more direct evaluation of the unique contributions of the various interventions, like parent participation, to the overall outcomes of reducing student alcohol use. Nor were we able to assess a dose-response effect for the parent interventions or examine the differential quality of the parents' implementation of Project Northland suggestions. These are all topics for future research.

PowerLines. Like the Amazing Alternatives! Program, the eighth grade PowerLines intervention primarily took place in the classroom in eight sessions, typically conducted over a four week period. It was designed to introduce students to groups within their communities that might influence underage drinking. Small group projects were used in which students had direct interviews in person or by the telephone with community leaders. The students presented their findings and suggestions to their classmates and school administrators about ways to solve the problem of underage drinking in their communities. Much less effort was devoted to the parent intervention in eighth grade, as the intervention strategy was to focus on the peer group and social environment outside the family.

Parents continued to receive the newsletter, *Northland Notes for Parents*; had opportunities to volunteer as adult facilitators for the peer-led alternative activities (Komro et al., 1994); and could participate in the community task forces. Since this was the third year for parent involvement programs to prevent underage drinking in our communities, the innovative strategy of using live theater, suggested by Safer and Harding (1993), was selected as a new vehicle for engaging parents and their eighth grade students. We initiated a collaboration with the Child's Play Theater Company of Minneapolis. Child's Play Theater offers an outreach program which uses actor-educators to work with students to produce guided improvisational theatrical productions that address a variety of social issues. Parents were invited to attend the performance, although attendance records were not feasible.

"It's My Party" was a collaborative effort between Project Northland and Child's Play Theater that evolved into a "tour" of northeastern Minnesota in March, 1994, through the Project Northland intervention communities. The tour consisted of two teams of actor-educators who were trained to conduct a three and one-half hour workshop with 10 selected eighth grade students from each of the 20 intervention schools. Following the workshop, and on the same day, these students performed the play for their peers, parents, and members of the community.

"It's My Party" was a melodrama set in the 1950s involving an adult character named Jack who arrived in town to promote an alcohol product to teens in the community using peer pressure and the latest advertising tricks. The story was relayed by a present day mother to her teen-aged daughter who was planning a party. The play allowed the teen actors to model to their audience of peers and parents many of the themes from previous years including parent-child communication about alcohol, family rules and consequences against underage drinking, resisting peer pressure and media influences to use, and ways parents and teens can plan alcohol-free popular and fun events. The play was well received in the intervention communities, attended by approximately 2,700 people in 20 performances. As with the Slick Tracy characters and themes, the play had inherent appeal with this age group and was discussed fondly in subsequent program years.

LESSONS FROM PROJECT NORTHLAND

The first phase of Project Northland demonstrated that it was feasible to implement multi-level community-wide programs based on behavioral theory in a large number of communities with successful implementation and high participation levels and resulting lower rates of drinking by the intervention subjects (Komro et al., 1994; Perry et al., 1996; Toomey et al., 1997; Williams et al., 1995). We demonstrated very high participation rates among students, including those who were higher risk, their parents, their teachers, and community members. Use of such approaches in rural and small town American communities with high alcohol use rates can significantly delay onset and reduce alcohol use at least until eighth grade. Cigarette, marijuana, and poly-drug use were also significantly reduced in baseline non-users in the intervention group. The interventions also changed a number of psychosocial factors related to underage drinking, including increased parent communication about rules and consequences for underage drinking. We did have less success in changing the larger social environment in Phase 1 with access to alcohol remaining too high. Changing the larger social environment that supports older teen drinking by reducing access to alcohol with interventions targeted at merchants and other adults, and changing norms that support drinking by older adolescents, as well as convincing high school students that alcohol does not have to be a prominent feature of their social lives, are our challenges for Phase 2.

Our study design does not allow us to tease out the relative effectiveness of the various program components. To be able to do so would have required a prohibitively costly sample size. However, we are confident that the parent components described in this paper were key ingredients for our program's effectiveness. This assumption is based on our theoretical framework that was informed by empirical research from over the last 20 years completed by ourselves and others, as well as practical experience in implementing Project Northland programs with approximately 1,200 young adolescents and their parents (Toomey et al., 1997; Williams et al., 1995).

The success of Project Northland in delaying the onset of drinking during early adolescence, reducing targeted risk factors (e.g., peer influence to drink), and increasing targeted protective factors (e.g., parent communication about rules and consequences) could not have been accomplished without the successful implementation of our programs. Durlak (1998) suggested some of the ingredients for successful program implementation that we also found crucial for Project Northland's effectiveness. The six months to one year period for developing and testing our programs allowed us to carefully evaluate and change the programs as needed. Even though several of the Project Northland programs were based on previous work, our pilot tests frequently revealed that various components either did not work as intended or suggested ways to substantially improve the materials. The first draft of the sixth grade activity books, where Slick Tracy, Breathtest Mahoney, and others were drawn as adults, provides an example. After the first pilot test, students in focus groups told us that they overwhelmingly preferred having characters their same age. We were fortunate to have the resources to redraw and rewrite the scripts based on input from young adolescents about how to make the materials more appealing. Talking with, listening to, and observing young adolescents, their parents, and teachers provided innumerable opportunities to improve our materials by making them more relevant to our target audiences, which likely contributed to our high participation rates.

Having Project Northland coordinators assigned to each of our schools, and a full-time staff member to coordinate program implementation across the schools, were also essential to ensure effective program implementation. Teacher training was another essential ingredient, and was not relegated to a few minutes of volunteer staff time. Rather, teachers were brought together from across school districts and trained during full and half-day sessions. The training occurred during school hours and schools were reimbursed by the project for substitute teachers.

Finally, we are fortunate to have a multi-disciplinary staff with many years experience working together to develop health promotion programs for youth. The cumulative experience of working together on many different public health interventions has made us sensitive to pitfalls to avoid in program implementation. If the field of primary prevention is to advance, stable funding for continued multi-disciplinary research, ever more elusive, remains essential.

NOTE

1. Many people contributed to the successful development and implementation of the early adolescent interventions for Project Northland: Bonnie Dudovitz (writer and curriculum specialist); Sara Veblen-Mortenson (intervention coordinator); Glenn Quist (consultant and graphic artist); Rebecca Turner (desktop publishing); Traci Toomey (7th grade home program); Kelli Komro (7th grade peer program); and the local community coordinators responsible for implementing our programs in the schools (Tom Burman, Lynette Eck, Kathy Lingren, Judy Lundquist, Russell Maki, James Pavlek, Peter Pierson, and Sue Wetschka). We are also grateful to the teachers, staff, students, and parents from Fitzgerald Middle School, Mankato, Minnesota, for participating in multiple pilot tests of our interventions. The authors have previously acknowledged, and remain ever appreciative, of the contributions of their subjects: the school districts, students, and parents in northeastern Minnesota participating in Project Northland research. Project Northland is funded by the National Institute on Alcohol Abuse and Alcoholism (R01-AA08596; R01-AA10719).

REFERENCES

Ary, D.V., Tildesley, E., Hops, H. & Andrews, J. (1993). The influence of parent, sibling, and peer modeling in attitudes on adolescent use of alcohol. *The International Journal of Addictions*, *28*(9), 853-880.

Botvin, G.J., Schinke, S.P., & Orlandi, M.S. (1989). Psycho-social approaches to substance abuse prevention: Theoretical foundations and empirical findings. *Crisis: International Journal of Suicide and Crisis Studies, 10*, 62-77.

Brook, J.S., Whiteman, M., Gordon, A.S., Nomura, C., & Brook, D.W. (1986). Onset of adolescent drinking: A longitudinal study of intrapersonal and interpersonal antecedents. In B. Stimmel (Ed.), *Alcohol and substance abuse in women and children*. New York: The Haworth Press, Inc.

Dryfoos, J.G. (1993). Preventing substance use: Rethinking strategies. *American Journal of Public Health, 83*, 793-795.

Durlak, J. (1998). Why program implementation is important. *Journal of Prevention & Intervention in the Community, 17*(2), 5-18.

Harding, W.M., Apsler, R., & Walsh, W.A. (1989). *Identification of parental program structures for deterring adolescent drinking and driving. Vol. II: Literature Review.* (DOT HS 807 556). Washington, DC: U.S. Department of Transportation.

Johnston, L.D., O'Malley, P.M., Bachman, J.G. (1993). *National Survey Results on Drug Use from the Monitoring the Future Study, 1975-1992 (Vol. I: Secondary School Students)* Rockville, MD: National Institute on Drug Abuse.

Klitzner, M., Gruenewald, P.J., & Bamberger, E. (1990). The assessment of parent-lead prevention programs: A preliminary assessment of impact. *Journal of Drug Education, 20*, 77-94.

Komro, K.A., Perry, C.L., Veblen-Mortenson, S., & Williams, C.L. (1994). Peer participation in Project Northland: A community-wide alcohol use prevention project. *Journal of School Health, 64*, 318-322.

National Institute on Alcohol Abuse and Alcoholism (1991). County alcohol problem indicators, 1979-1985. *U.S. Alcohol Epidemiologic Data Reference Manual (Vol. 3)*. Rockville, MD: NIAAA.

National Institute on Alcohol Abuse and Alcoholism (1994). *Eighth special report to the U.S. Congress on alcohol and health* (NIH Publ. No. 94-3699). Washington, DC: U.S. Department of Health and Human Services.

Pentz, M.A., Dwyer, J.H., MacKinnon, D.P., Flay, B.R., Hansen, W.B., Wang, E.Y.I., & Johnson, C.A. (1989). A multicommunity trail for primary prevention of adolescent drug abuse: Effects on drug use prevalence. *Journal of the American Medical Association, 261*(22), 3259-3266.

Perry, C.L., Crockett, S.J., & Pirie, P. (1987). Influencing parental health behavior: Implications of community assessments. *Health Education, 18*, 68-77.

Perry, C.L., Luepker, R.V., Murray, D.M., Hearn, M.D., Halper, A., Dudovitz, B., Maile, M.C., & Smyth, M. (1989). Parent involvement with children's health promotion: A one-year follow-up of the Minnesota home team. *Health Education Quarterly, 16*(2), 171-180.

Perry, C.L., Williams, C.L., Forster, J.L., Wolfson, M., Wagenaar A.C., Finnegan, J.R., McGovern, P.G., Veblen-Mortenson, S., Komro, K.A., & Anstine, P.S. (1993). Background, conceptualization, and design of a community-wide research program on adolescent alcohol use: Project Northland. *Health Education Research: Theory & Practice, 8*(1), 125-136.

Perry, C.L., Williams, C.L., Veblen-Mortenson, S., Toomey, T., Komro, K., Anstine, P.S., McGovern, P., Finnegan, J.R., Forster, J.L., Wagenaar, A.C., & Wolfson, M. (1996). Outcomes of a community-wide alcohol use prevention program during early adolescence: Project Northland. *American Journal of Public Health*, *86*(7), 956-965.

Peterson, P.L., Hawkins, J.D., Abbott, R.D., Catalano, R.F. (1994). Disentangling the effects of parental drinking, family management, and parental alcohol norms on current drinking by black and white adolescents. *Journal of Research on Adolescents*, *4*(2), 203-227.

Safer, L.A., & Harding, C.G. (1993). Under pressure program: Using live theater to investigate adolescents' attitudes and behavior related to drug and alcohol abuse education and prevention. *Adolescence*, *28*, 135-148.

Thomas, B.S. (1992). Patterns of alcohol and other drug use in an Iowa community. *Journal of School Health*, *62*, 454-458.

Toomey, T.L., Williams, C.L., Perry, C.L., Murray, D.M., Dudovitz, B., & Veblen-Mortenson, S. (1997). An alcohol primary prevention program for parents of 7th graders: The amazing alternatives! Home program. *Journal of Child & Adolescent Substance Abuse*, *5*(4), 35-53.

Trends in drug and alcohol use by youth in the USA. (1993, July-Sept.) *Statistical Bulletin*, *74*, 19-27.

Wagenaar, A.C., & Perry, C.L. (1994). Community strategies for the reduction of youth drinking: Theory and application. *Journal of Research on Adolescence*, *4*, 319-345.

Werch, C.E., Young, M., Clark, M., Garrett, C., Hooks, S., & Kersten, C. (1991). Effects of a take-home drug prevention program on drug-related communication and beliefs of parents and children. *Journal of School Health*, *61*(8), 346-350.

Williams, C.L., Perry, C.L., Dudovitz, B., Veblen-Mortenson, S., Anstine, P.S., Komro, K.A., & Toomey, T.L. (1995). A home-based prevention program for sixth grade alcohol use: Results from Project Northland. *Journal of Primary Prevention*, *16*(2), 125-147.

Some Exemplars of Implementation

Joseph A. Durlak
Loyola University Chicago

Joseph R. Ferrari
DePaul University

SUMMARY. Several successful prevention programs are recognized as exemplars of implementation. Complicated multidimensional interventions with different goals and directed at different target populations have been conducted with a high degree of fidelity using a common set of strategies. Future research priorities involve identifying the specific factors that promote implementation and determining what levels of implementation are necessary to achieve maximum program impact. *[Article copies available for a fee from The Haworth Document Delivery Service: 1-800-342-9678. E-mail address: getinfo@haworth.com]*

Because implementation plays such an important role in interventions, this paper discusses a few exemplars. The intent is to credit some researchers who have been successful in program implementation, offer additional references for interested readers to pursue, and then, in a brief final section, to present a few questions for future researchers. The discussion of good examples of program implementation begins with the contributors to this volume.

Address correspondence to: Joseph A. Durlak, Department of Psychology, Loyola University Chicago, 6525 North Sheridan Road, Chicago, IL 60626.

[Haworth co-indexing entry note]: "Some Exemplars of Implementation." Durlak, Joseph A., and Joseph R. Ferrari. Co-published simultaneously in *Journal of Prevention & Intervention in the Community* (The Haworth Press, Inc.) Vol. 17, No. 2, 1998, pp. 81-89; and: *Program Implementation in Preventive Trials* (ed: Joseph A. Durlak, and Joseph R. Ferrari) The Haworth Press, Inc., 1998, pp. 81-89. Single or multiple copies of this article are available for a fee from The Haworth Document Delivery Service [1-800-342-9678, 9:00 a.m. - 5:00 p.m. (EST). E-mail address: getinfo@haworthpressinc.com].

ADOLESCENT DEPRESSION

Clarke (this volume) reported very good to excellent levels of implementation in four studies (mean levels of at least 78%) with little variability across change agents except in the first trial. In fact, a few group leaders received perfect scores for fidelity which is quite unusual. The highly structured nature of the intervention and the use of manuals to guide the change agents seem to be major factors contributing to the good fidelity attained in these studies.

Although Clarke bemoaned the fact that the mediating effects of implementation on outcomes could not be observed because of the high and consistent fidelity that was achieved, this is a "problem" that many researchers would be glad to have. It is noteworthy that even though fidelity was high in the initial 1990 study discussed by Clarke, it did increase in subsequent studies (from an initial mean of 78% to 93% in the targeted prevention study). Repeated experience with an intervention seems to help the implementation process because it gives investigators opportunities to fine-tune an intervention and to learn how to help others deliver the program more effectively.

Clarke also presented some internal consistency and interjudge reliability data on a 10-item fidelity scale. This is valuable information; the former data are frequently missing from implementation studies. Investigators who devise implementation scales to monitor their interventions should assess their psychometric properties. Internal consistency might need improvement because there might be more dimensions to implementation than anticipated.

SANKOFA

Hines, Macias and Perrino (this volume) provided a nice example of an intervention culturally tailored to urban African-American youth. SANKOFA draws upon African traditions and fables and also incorporates current media to make the program highly relevant for young people. Hines et al. solicited input from adolescents in order to make the program as engaging as possible. Their experiences also highlight the importance of being flexible in program scheduling; they found it impossible to conduct an after-school program as initially planned and eventually administered their intervention during school hours although this too presented them with difficulties. Another nice feature of this intervention was that it was offered not only to students in regular high schools but also to those in juvenile detention centers, alternative schools for behaviorally disordered youth, and to community-based organizations serving high school dropouts. These latter groups are often overlooked in preventive interventions which tend to target the most easily accessible populations. Preliminary findings suggested SANKOFA was equally effective across different sites.

RCMHC

Lynch, Geller, Hunt, Galano and Dubas (this volume) also reported very good to excellent levels of implementation, means of 77% for quantity and 82% for quality (which they called content and approach respectively). Remarkably, there was also a 100% return rate for the 420 lesson forms that teachers had to complete in order to monitor program implementation. It is obvious that a good working relationship was established with school staff.

Lynch et al. attributed much of their success to their use of a participatory research strategy. Teachers learned the importance of careful program evaluation and their input into the program and competence in school settings were respected. Lynch et al. also made the interesting observation that teachers who lacked good classroom management skills seemed to have more trouble implementing the intervention. This observation suggests that good implementation may be dependent on the presence of other skills that may have to be developed before new interventions can be well implemented which would increase the pressures and responsibilities for trainers and supervisors. Another possible implication is that some change agents may not be able to develop the proficiency necessary to mount new complicated interventions (either out of lack of motivation or lack of competence). For classroom-level interventions such as RCMHC it means that the intervention might never reach all classrooms. For interventions attempting systematic change at the school level, however, there is the question of what proportion of school staff must be involved to achieve effective organizational change. Data are not currently available regarding the "critical mass" needed for systemic school changes.

PROJECT NORTHLAND

Williams and Perry (this volume) reported that 90% of parents completed at least some of the 6th grade Project Northland booklets and that 75% completed most of them. This level of parent participation is exceptional in prevention. For instance, both the rate and intensity of parent involvement are important and no preventionists have reported that all eligible parents have attended all program sessions and completed all activities. It is not uncommon for less than 20% of eligible parents to participate in prevention programs (Baranowski et al., 1990; Cohen & Rice, 1995; Spoth & Redmond, 1994); participation rates around 50% are often difficult to attain, and rates above 60% are unusual (Crockett, Mullis, Perry, & Luepker, 1989; Rohrbach et al., 1994; Spoth & Redmond, 1994; Weeks et al., 1997). There are fewer data on the intensity of parental participation. It is not atypical for parents, however, to attend less than half of scheduled meetings or complete only half of requested activities (Baranowski et al. 1990; Dumka, Garza, Roosa & Stoerzinger, 1997; Spoth & Redmond, 1994), which is why the Project Northland data are exceptional.

Williams and Perry took the straightforward approach of asking parents for their preferences and accommodating their wishes as much as possible. Few parents wish to attend evening meetings at school or in the community (Perry, Crockett & Pirie, 1987). The most successful strategy of involving parents in school-based programs has been to devise some type of home-based parent component (Durlak, 1997). Usually, this is a school curriculum that requires parent involvement in the completion of the child's homework. These parent-child activities vary as a function of the program. In drug abuse prevention, the parent might be required to assist in role play situations in which the child practices assertiveness or refusal skills (i.e., how to say "no" effectively; Rohrbach et al., 1994). In other cases, children and parents evaluate the nutritional value of foods available at home (Crockett et al., 1989). In some programs, children receive reinforcement at school in relation to how many activities their parents complete with them, which probably motivates more parents to become more involved.

In other areas of prevention, staff who make home visits (compared to asking parents to come to clinics or community centers) have been successful in promoting the physical health and development of children born to young mothers (Olds & Kitzman, 1993). Another effective approach has been to develop videos for family use at home to improve communication and discussion about HIV/AIDS (Winett & Anderson, 1994). Home-based parent components avoid the many practical problems associated with attending meetings at school or in the community. School meetings can work, however, if they are scheduled at times the parents indicate are most convenient to them and if needed child care and transportation are provided (Dumka et al., 1997).

ADDITIONAL EXEMPLARS

Several programs that achieved good levels of implementation were cited elsewhere (see Durlak, Table 2, this volume). Two additional programs deserve attention because of the scope, intensity and success of their implementation efforts.

CATCH

CATCH (Child and Adolescent Trial for Cardiovascular Health) was the largest and most sophisticated randomized controlled school health education intervention ever conducted (see special journal issues devoted to CATCH edited by Resnicow, Robinson & Frank, 1996; Stone, 1994). CATCH was a 3-year longitudinal study involving over 5,000 ethically diverse 3rd graders drawn from 96 schools in four states. The program was successful in improving several facets of children's cardiovascular health through a multi component intervention that included a classroom-based social skills curriculum, parent participation, school policy initiatives, and organizational changes in schools' physical education and school lunch programs. The major goals were to modify students' diet, level of physical activity and smoking.

The planning and resources devoted to implementation were impressive. First, there were designated staff with primary responsibility for program implementation. Second, initial training of school staff was supplemented by follow-up consultation, and booster training and make-up training sessions were scheduled in the case of absences. Third, observational procedures used to assess implementation were field-checked for their feasibility, reliability and validity, and modified as necessary before they were formally introduced into the program. Fourth, the monitoring and assessment of the implementation of different program components was both intensive and extensive.

For example, monthly visits indicated that school food service staff were correctly following 90% of 30 specific guidelines related to menu planning, food purchase, food preparation, and program promotion (e.g., following recipes using standardized measuring utensils). Extensive classroom observations indicated that 88% of the classroom curriculum was completed with good integrity. Part of the classroom curriculum required parental participation to help children complete homework assignments. Parents participated in 67% of the possible activities. Six randomly selected week-long observations indicated that teachers successfully implemented most of the elements of the newly prescribed physical education classes. Program schools were also asked to change their tobacco policies to create totally smoke-free environments (no smoking permitted by visitors, staff or students at any time during the school day and at any school-related functions). The percentage of program schools that developed the desired smoke-free policies increased from 45% at pre to 78% at the end of the 3-year period.

Although technically not part of program implementation, CATCH staff also monitored the extent to which participating students reported that peers, teachers and parents supported their efforts at behavioral change. Program students perceived significantly more support over time from significant others for choosing healthy foods but not for increasing their levels of vigorous physical exercise. These findings are important in suggesting in what ways children's social environment had or had not changed to reinforce CATCH goals.

High/Scope

In another ambitious project, the High/Scope Educational Research Foundation of Ypsilanti, Michigan embarked on a series of multi year evaluations of inservice training of early childhood educators (summarized in Epstein, 1993). This project, called the Training of Trainers (TOT) Evaluation, was so successful that by the end of 1991, 80 projects had trained over 1,000 consultants who, in turn, had trained an estimated 26,000 teachers who were working with approximately one-quarter of a million preschool children annually.

Staff were disseminating the High/Scope preschool curriculum which outcome research has confirmed is one of the most effective approaches to preschool education. Participants in this preschool curriculum have continued to demonstrate numerous educational and social benefits 25 years after their participation and the High/Scope program is cost effective, returning over $8.00 in benefits for every dollar spent (Barnett, 1993). Therefore, it is important to document that this program can be effectively incorporated into other settings.

In their evaluations focusing on program implementation, data were drawn from 244 programs in which newly-trained teachers were using the High/Scope curriculum compared to 122 comparison programs (Epstein, 1993). Independent observations of teaching practices were conducted by 25 raters who achieved a high level of reliability in their observations (89.5%) and who were kept blind to the teacher's experimental condition (High/Scope or comparison). Data indicated that teachers implemented the High/Scope program with a high degree of fidelity; ratings averaged 4.02

on a 5-point scale. Outcome data indicated that children in High/Scope programs were significantly superior to comparison children in initiative, social relations, and cognitive and motor development and there was a significant relationship obtained between the level of program implementation and children's development. TOT is an impressive demonstration because it occurred at a level "once-removed" from the original High/Scope program. That is, High/Scope staff were able to train preschool educators who in turn effectively trained others in how to replicate the curriculum. Therefore, TOT findings indicate that it is possible to disseminate a validated preschool curriculum into many different settings.

Factors Affecting Implementation

All the interventions discussed here are complicated multidimensional programs making it impossible to identify how different practices contributed to better implementation. It is notable, however, that each program followed the strategies outlined earlier (Durlak, this volume). That is, authors: (a) used a theory-driven intervention that allowed them to clearly specify its main features; (b) collaborated with members of the host community (including teachers, students and parents) prior to the intervention to secure their input and commitment; (c) carefully trained change agents and provided ongoing supervision and consultation after the program began; (d) were prepared to deal with unexpected problems; (e) did pilot work to test their interventions and/or implementation methods; and (f) designated staff who had responsibilities for implementation. Additional strategies were used depending on local circumstances. It is perhaps no coincidence that two contributors (Lynch et al., this volume; Hines et al., this volume) had formal written agreements with host agencies. These agreements seemed to strengthen the host agency's commitment to the project and clarified the responsibilities of evaluators and field staff.

FUTURE RESEARCH DIRECTIONS

Experience indicates that complicated multidimensional interventions can be conducted with a high degree of fidelity if sufficient time and attention are devoted to the many issues affecting program implementation. Regardless of the area of prevention, the target population, and program features and mechanics, most have used a common set of strategies to promote implementation. Research on implementation is in its relative infancy, however, and there is still much to be learned. For instance, several questions need to be addressed in future research:

1. What levels of implementation quantity and quality are necessary for maximum program impact?
2. How do different factors influence implementation?
3. What percentage of target groups such as teachers, parents and community-based organizations elect to participate in preventive interventions and what factors are associated with their participation?
4. How can the rate and intensity of involvement be improved for different groups?

REFERENCES

Baranowski, T., Simons-Morton, B., Hooks, P., Henske, J., Tiernan, K., Dunn, J. K., Burkhalter, H., Harper, J., & Palmer, J. (1990). A center-based program for exercise change among Black American families. *Health Education Quarterly*, *17*, 179-196.

Barnett, W. S. (1993). Benefit-cost analysis of preschool education: Findings from a 25-year follow-up. *American Journal of Orthopsychiatry*, 500-508.

Cohen, D. A., & Rice, J. C. (1995). A parent-targeted intervention for adolescent substance use prevention: Lessons learned. *Evaluation Review*, *1995*, 159-180.

Crockett, S. J., Mullis, R., Perry, C. L., & Luepker, R. V. (1989). Parent education in youth-directed nutrition intervention. *Preventive Medicine*, *18*, 475-491.

Dumka, L. E., Garza, C. A., Roosa, M. W., & Stoerzinger, H. D. (1997). Recruitment and retention of high-risk families into a preventive parent training intervention. *Journal of Primary Prevention*, *18*, 25-39.

Durlak, J. A. (1997). *Successful prevention programs for children and adolescents*. New York: Plenum.

Epstein, A. S. (1993). *Training for Quality: Improving early childhood programs through systematic inservice training*. Monograph #9 of the High/Scope Educational Research Foundation. Ypsilanti, MI: High/Scope Press.

Olds, D. L., & Kitzman, H. (1993). Review of research on home visiting for pregnant women and parents of young children. *The Future of Children*, *3*, 53-92.

Perry, C. L.,, Crockett, S. J., & Pirie, P. (1987). Influencing parental health behavior: Implications of community assessments. *Health Education*, *18*, 68-77.

Resnicow, K., Robinson, T. N., & Frank, E. (Eds.). (1996). The multicenter Child and Adolescent Trial for Cardiovascular Health (CATCH): Promoting cardiovascular health through schools. [Special issue]. *Preventive Medicine*, *25*(4).

Rohrbach, L. A., Hodgson, C. S., Broder, B. I., Montgomery, S. B., Flay, B. R., Hansen, W. B., & Pentz, M. A. (1994). Parental participation in drug abuse prevention: Results from the Midwestern Prevention Project. *Journal of Research on Adolescence*, *4*, 295-317.

Spoth, R., & Redmond, C. (1994). Effective recruitment of parents into family-focused prevention research: A comparison of two strategies. *Health Psychology*, *9*, 353-370.

Stone, E. J. (Ed.). (1994). Process evaluation in the multicenter Child and Adolescent Trial for Cardiovascular Health (CATCH) [Special issue]. *Health Education Quarterly*; Suppl. 2: S3-143.

Weeks, K., Levy, S. R., Gordon, A. K., Handler, A., Perhats, C., & Flay, B. R. (1997). Does parental involvement make a difference? The impact of parent interactive activities on students in a school-based AIDS prevention program. *AIDS Education and Prevention*, *9*, Suppl. A, 90-106.

Winett, R. A., & Anderson, E. S. (1994). HIV prevention in youth: A framework for research and action. In T. H. Ollendick & R. J. Prinz (Eds.), *Advances in clinical child psychology* (Vol. 16, pp. 1-43). New York: Plenum.

Index